CO-ASA-695

Curbside
Consultation
in Pediatric Infectious Disease

49 Clinical Questions

CURBSIDE CONSULTATION IN PEDIATRICS
SERIES

SERIES EDITOR, LISA B. ZAOUTIS, MD

Curbside
Consultation
in Pediatric Infectious Disease

49 Clinical Questions

Angela L. Myers, MD, MPH, FAAP

Assistant Professor of Pediatrics
Section of Infectious Diseases
Pediatric Infectious Diseases Fellowship Program Director
Children's Mercy Hospitals & Clinics
University of Missouri-Kansas City School of Medicine
Kansas City, Kansas

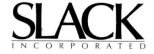

SLACK
INCORPORATED

www.Healio.com/books

ISBN: 978-1-61711-001-6

The procedures and practices described in this publication should be implemented in a manner consistent with the professional standards set for the circumstances that apply in each specific situation. Every effort has been made to confirm the accuracy of the information presented and to correctly relate generally accepted practices. The authors, editors, and publisher cannot accept responsibility for errors or exclusions or for the outcome of the material presented herein. There is no expressed or implied warranty of this book or information imparted by it. Care has been taken to ensure that drug selection and dosages are in accordance with currently accepted/recommended practice. Off-label uses of drugs may be discussed. Due to continuing research, changes in government policy and regulations, and various effects of drug reactions and interactions, it is recommended that the reader carefully review all materials and literature provided for each drug, especially those that are new or not frequently used. Some drugs or devices in this publication have clearance for use in a restricted research setting by the Food and Drug and Administration or FDA. Each professional should determine the FDA status of any drug or device prior to use in their practice.

Any review or mention of specific companies or products is not intended as an endorsement by the author or publisher.

SLACK Incorporated uses a review process to evaluate submitted material. Prior to publication, educators or clinicians provide important feedback on the content that we publish. We welcome feedback on this work.

Published by: SLACK Incorporated
                 6900 Grove Road
                 Thorofare, NJ 08086 USA
                 Telephone: 856-848-1000
                 Fax: 856-848-6091
                 www.Healio.com/books

Contact SLACK Incorporated for more information about other books in this field or about the availability of our books from distributors outside the United States.

Library of Congress Control Number: 2012932271
Curbside consultation in pediatric infectious disease : 49 clinical questions / [edited by] Angela L. Myers.
    p. ; cm. -- (Curbside consultation in pediatrics series)
  Pediatric infectious disease
  Includes bibliographical references and index.
   ISBN 978-1-61711-001-6 (pbk. : alk. paper)
   I. Myers, Angela L., 1977- II. Title: Pediatric infectious disease. III. Series: Curbside consultation in pediatrics series.
   [DNLM: 1. Communicable Diseases--therapy. 2. Child. 3. Communicable Diseases--diagnosis. 4. Infant. WC 100]
   Lc classification not assigned
   618.92'9--dc23
                      2012014867

Printed in the United States of America.

Last digit is print number: 10 9 8 7 6 5 4 3 2 1

Dedication

To Dave, Jackson, and Emma. You are my inspiration and the light of my life. I am eternally grateful for each and every day I have with you.

And to my parents, for always believing in who I would become.

Contents

Dedication .... *v*

Acknowledgments .... *xiii*

About the Editor .... *xv*

Contributing Authors .... *xvii*

Preface .... *xix*

Foreword by Janet R. Gilsdorf, MD .... *xxi*

Introduction .... *xxiii*

Section I **Urinary Tract Infection** 1

Question 1   Is It Appropriate to Treat a Suspected Urinary Tract Infection
Based on an In-Office Urine Dipstick Result, or Should the Specimen
Be Sent for Culture? Does the Age of the Patient Have Anything to Do
With the Decision? 3
Rene VanDeVoorde, MD

Question 2   When Should You Attempt to Obtain a Catheter Specimen Versus a
Clean Catch Specimen in the Setting of a Suspected Urinary Tract
Infection? 9
Rene VanDeVoorde, MD

Question 3   When Is Imaging, Such as Voiding Cystourethrogram and Renal
Ultrasound, Necessary for Children With a First Urinary Tract
Infection? 13
Rene VanDeVoorde, MD

Question 4   Is Prophylaxis Recommended for All Patients With
Vesicoureteral Reflux? 17
Rene VanDeVoorde, MD

Section II **Methicillin-Resistant *Staphylococcus aureus*** 21

Question 5   When Is Oral Antibiotic Therapy Necessary in the Setting
of Recurrent Methicillin-Resistant *Staphylococcus aureus*
Skin Infection/Boils? 23
Emily A. Thorell, MD

Question 6   Are Bleach Baths or Chlorhexidine Plus Mupirocin Ointment Useful to
Decolonize Patients With Recurrent Methicillin-Resistant *Staphylococcus
aureus* Infections? What Topical Recommendations Are Useful for
Patients With Recurrent Infections?..27
Emily A. Thorell, MD

Question 7   In What Settings Is Methicillin-Resistant *Staphylococcus
aureus* Spread?...31
Emily A. Thorell, MD

Question 8   Are There Environmental Cleaning or Personal Hygiene Interventions
That Can Be Used to Reduce Recurrences of Methicillin-Resistant
Staphylococcus aureus Infections?...35
Emily A. Thorell, MD

Section III   Tinea Capitis **39**

Question 9   How Long Does Tinea Capitis Need to Be Treated in Order
to Be Sure the Infection Has Cleared?..41
Jennifer Goldman, MD and Susan Abdel-Rahman, PharmD

Question 10   What Are the Methods by Which Tinea Capitis Can Be
Spread From Person to Person? 45
Jennifer Goldman, MD and Susan Abdel-Rahman, PharmD

Question 11   Do There Need to Be Visible Lesions to Diagnose Tinea Capitis?.............47
Jennifer Goldman, MD and Susan Abdel-Rahman, PharmD

Question 12   What Organisms Are Responsible for Causing Tinea Capitis?..................51
Jennifer Goldman, MD and Susan Abdel-Rahman, PharmD

Section IV   Tick-Borne Illness **53**

Question 13   What Are the Best Prophylactic Measures to Tell Families
to Use to Prevent Tick Bites? At What Age Are Agents Such as
DEET and Picaridin Safe to Use?..55
Kimberly C. Martin, DO and José R. Romero, MD, FAAP

Question 14   When Are Tick-Borne Infections Typically Seen in the
United States, and When Does the Peak Time Occur? 59
Kimberly C. Martin, DO and José R. Romero, MD, FAAP

Question 15   What Is the Best Empiric and/or Prophylactic Therapy
for a Child in Whom You Suspect a Tick-Borne Infection?.........................65
Kimberly C. Martin, DO and José R. Romero, MD, FAAP

Question 16   In What Parts of the United States Is Lyme Disease Seen, How Is
Diagnosis Confirmed, and What Is the Appropriate Treatment?..............69
Kimberly C. Martin, DO and José R. Romero, MD, FAAP

Section V   Atypical Pneumonia **75**

Question 17   Can You Make a Diagnosis of Atypical Pneumonia by Clinical
Presentation or Is Laboratory Evaluation Required? 77
Christopher R. Cannavino, MD

Question 18   What Are the Most Common Ages, Presenting Symptoms, and Common Organisms Associated With Cases of Atypical Pneumonia?..81
Christopher R. Cannavino, MD

Section VI Otitis Media..**85**

Question 19   What Is the Recommended Specific Treatment of Otitis Media Due to Multidrug-Resistant Pneumococcus? 87
Christopher J. Harrison, MD

Question 20   When Should Middle Ear Effusion Fluid Be Obtained?............93
Christopher J. Harrison, MD

Question 21   What Do You Do for a Patient Who Has Ear Tubes and Has Continuous Ear Drainage? 97
Christopher J. Harrison, MD

Question 22   What Is the Recommended Specific Treatment of Acute Otitis Media Due to Multidrug-Resistant Pneumococcus?.....................101
Christopher J. Harrison, MD

Section VII Pharyngitis..**107**

Question 23   Is a Throat Culture Necessary in the Setting of a Negative Rapid Streptococcal Antigen Test?............................109
Kevin B. Spicer, MD, PhD, MPH and Preeti Jaggi, MD

Question 24   What Is the Best Treatment Option for Group A Streptococcal Pharyngitis? What if the Patient Is Allergic to Beta-Lactam Antibiotics? 113
Kevin B. Spicer, MD, PhD, MPH and Preeti Jaggi, MD

Question 25   Why Do We Treat Streptococcal Pharyngitis When It Is a Self-Limited Illness? 117
Kevin B. Spicer, MD, PhD, MPH; Preeti Jaggi, MD; and Angela L. Myers, MD, MPH, FAAP

Question 26   Should I Treat the Asymptomatic Siblings of the Patient Who Has a Positive Rapid Streptococcal Antigen Test? 123
Kevin B. Spicer, MD, PhD, MPH; Preeti Jaggi, MD; and Angela L. Myers, MD, MPH, FAAP

Question 27   What Are the Best Clinical Indicators That My Patient May Have Streptococcal Pharyngitis?..127
Kevin B. Spicer, MD, PhD, MPH and Preeti Jaggi, MD

Section VIII Viral Testing **131**

Question 28 How Sensitive and Specific Are the Office-Based Rapid
Respiratory Syncytial Virus and Rapid Influenza Tests? 133
Rebecca C. Brady, MD

Question 29 If I Have a 3-Month-Old Infant in the Office With Respiratory
Symptoms and Negative Viral Testing, Should I Proceed With a
Sepsis Evaluation? 137
Archana Chatterjee, MD, PhD

Question 30 If I Have a 5-Week-Old Infant With Positive Rapid Viral Testing
Who Does Not Need Hospital Admission, Is a Sepsis
Evaluation Necessary? 141
Archana Chatterjee, MD, PhD

Section IX   Diarrhea **145**

Question 31 When Are Antibiotics Indicated for a Child With a Bacterial
Cause of Diarrhea? 147
Amber Hoffman, MD

Question 32 What Are Likely to Be the Most Common Viral Pathogens
Causing Diarrhea Since the Decrease in Rotavirus Cases
With Increase in Vaccine Uptake? 153
Amber Hoffman, MD

Section X   Upper Respiratory Tract Infection/Sinusitis **157**

Question 33 When Should I Be Worried About Immune Deficiency
in the Setting of Recurrent Upper Respiratory Tract Infections? 159
Adam L. Hersh, MD, PhD

Question 34 What Are the Most Common Viral Respiratory Pathogens
in Infants in the First Year of Life? 161
Adam L. Hersh, MD, PhD

Question 35 What Antibiotics Are Recommended Empirically for Acute Bacterial
Sinusitis in a Patient Who Has Not Received Antibiotics Recently? 165
Adam L. Hersh, MD, PhD

Question 36 What Antibiotics Are Recommended to Treat Acute Bacterial
Sinusitis in the Patient Who Had a Course of Amoxicillin
Within the Last Few Weeks for Otitis Media? 169
Adam L. Hersh, MD, PhD

Section XI Community-Acquired Pneumonia **173**

Question 37 What Is the Most Common Pathogen Involved in
Community-Acquired Pneumonia, and the Empiric
Therapy of Choice in the Preschool–Aged Child With Fever
to 102°F, Rales, and a Lobar Infiltrate on Chest Radiograph?................... 175
Christopher R. Cannavino, MD

Question 38 When Should Concern Arise About *Staphylococcus aureus* in a
Patient With Pneumonia? 179
Christopher R. Cannavino, MD

Section XII Epstein-Barr Virus/Cytomegalovirus **183**

Question 39 When Are Steroids Indicated in the Setting of Known Acute
Epstein-Barr Virus Infection?.. 185
Masako Shimamura, MD and Rebecca W. Widener, MD

Question 40 What Laboratory Test(s) Should Be Obtained in the
Setting of Suspected Congenital Cytomegalovirus Infection? 189
Masako Shimamura, MD and Rebecca W. Widener, MD

Question 41 When Should Serologic Testing Be Performed Instead of
a Monospot, and How Do I Interpret Results of Epstein-Barr
Virus Serologies?.. 193
Masako Shimamura, MD and Rebecca W. Widener, MD

Question 42 What Should I Tell a Pregnant Mother of a 2 Year Old
Who Has Recently Been Diagnosed With Congenital
Cytomegalovirus Infection About Her Risk for Developing
Infection as Well as Prevention Techniques? 197
Masako Shimamura, MD and Rebecca W. Widener, MD

Section XIII Lymphadenopathy..**201**

Question 43 A 13-Year-Old Female Presents With Symptoms of Cat Scratch
Disease. What Is the Best Approach to the Diagnosis and
the Preferred Management of a Patient With Cat
Scratch Disease? 203
Ankhi Dutta, MD, MPH and Debra L. Palazzi, MD

Question 44 What Are the Most Common Pathogens and Empiric Treatment(s)
of Choice in a Patient With Suspected Acute Bacterial
Lymphadenitis? 209
Ankhi Dutta, MD, MPH and Debra L. Palazzi, MD

Section XIV Prolonged Fever **213**

Question 45   What Is the Differential Diagnosis in a 3-Year-Old Female With a
7-Day History of Fever, Red Eyes and Lips, Rash, and
Swollen Hands? 215
Laura Patricia Stadler, MEd, MD, MS

Question 46   What Imaging Evaluation Should I Consider in an 11-Year-Old
Male With a 2-Week History of Fever and Complaints of
Low Back Pain and a Progressive Limp? 221
Laura Patricia Stadler, MEd, MD, MS

Section XV Candidiasis **225**

Question 47   A 5-Week-Old Infant Was Recently Diagnosed With Thrush and
Treated With Nystatin for 10 Days Without Improvement.
Should I Obtain a Culture of the Infant's Mucosa and Change
His Therapy? What Other Problems Should I Be Thinking
About in This Setting? 227
Amber Hoffman, MD

Section XVI Recurrent Fever **231**

Question 48   What Diagnostic Testing, If Any, Should Be Performed for a
Normally Developing Toddler Who Attends a Day Care Center,
Develops Frequent Fevers, and Commonly Has Respiratory
Tract Symptoms? What Is the Most Common Reason for This
Presentation? 233
Aimee Hersh, MD and Erica F. Lawson, MD

Question 49   A 2-Year-Old Patient Has Had Recurrent Fevers for the Last Year.
He Often Has a Red Throat, Adenopathy, and Stomatitis
With His Fevers. I Am Concerned About Periodic Fever, Aphthous
Stomatitis, Pharyngitis, and Cervical Adenitis Syndrome. What Are
the Treatment Options for This Diagnosis? 237
Aimee Hersh, MD and Erica F. Lawson, MD

Financial Disclosures 241
Index 243

Acknowledgments

I would like to acknowledge the following individuals for their contributions and dedication to this book: Carrie Kotlar, April Billick, Jason Newland, Christopher Harrison, Kristina Bryant, Laura Stadler, and—most of all—my mentor and friend, Mary Anne Jackson.

About the Editor

Angela L. Myers, MD, MPH, FAAP, is a board-certified pediatric infectious diseases physician and is currently an Assistant Professor of Pediatrics at the University of Missouri-Kansas City School of Medicine. She is the pediatric infectious diseases fellowship director at Children's Mercy Hospital & Clinics. Dr. Myers received her undergraduate and medical degree from the University of Missouri-Kansas City School of Medicine in the combined 6-year program, and completed her pediatrics residency and pediatric infectious diseases fellowship at Children's Mercy Hospitals & Clinics. Active in research, her main interests revolve around childhood and adult vaccine knowledge, attitudes, and beliefs, as well as using novel health information technologies to improve vaccination rates for influenza. She currently oversees several funded studies evaluating vaccine beliefs as well as implementation of various strategies to increase immunization rates of both children and adults. She is the author of 2 book questions and more than 15 publications in pediatric journals and is also actively involved in committee work for the Pediatric Infectious Diseases Society program training committee and the graduate medical education council at her affiliated medical school.

Contributing Authors

Susan Abdel-Rahman, PharmD (Questions 9, 10, 11, 12)
Division of Clinical Pharmacology and Medical Toxicology
Department of Pediatrics
The Children's Mercy Hospital and Clinics
Kansas City, Missouri

Rebecca C. Brady, MD (Question 28)
Associate Professor of Clinical Pediatrics
Cincinnati Children's Hospital Medical Center
Cincinnati, Ohio

Christopher R. Cannavino, MD (Questions 17, 18, 37, 38)
Divisions of Infectious Diseases & Hospital Medicine
Rady Children's Hospital—San Diego
Assistant Clinical Professor of Pediatrics
University of California at San Diego
Director, Pediatrics Clerkship
UCSD School of Medicine
San Diego, California

Archana Chatterjee, MD, PhD (Questions 29, 30)
Assistant Dean for Faculty Affairs
Chief, Division of Pediatric Infectious Diseases
Professor of Pediatrics
Creighton University School of Medicine
Omaha, Nebraska

Ankhi Dutta, MD, MPH (Questions 43, 44)
Pediatric Infectious Diseases
Brazos Valley Community Action Agency
College Station, Texas

Jennifer Goldman, MD (Questions 9, 10, 11, 12)
Pediatric Infectious Diseases/Clinical Pharmacology Fellow
Children's Mercy Hospital and Clinics
University of Missouri at Kansas City
Kansas City, Missouri

Christopher J. Harrison, MD (Questions 19, 20, 21, 22)
Director of ID Research Laboratory
Director of Pediatric VTEUC
Children's Mercy Hospitals and Clinics
Professor of Pediatrics
University of Missouri at Kansas City
Kansas City, Missouri

Adam L. Hersh, MD, PhD (Questions 33, 34, 35, 36)
Assistant Professor
Pediatric Infectious Diseases
University of Utah
Salt Lake City, Utah

Aimee Hersh, MD (Questions 48, 49)
Assistant Professor
University of Utah
Salt Lake City, Utah

Amber Hoffman, MD (Questions 31, 32, 47)
Assistant Professor of Pediatrics
University of Missouri at Kansas City School of Medicine
Associate Director, Pediatric Residency Program
Children's Mercy Hospitals & Clinics
Kansas City, Missouri

Preeti Jaggi, MD (Questions 23, 24, 25, 26, 27)
Assistant Professor of Pediatrics
Department of Infectious Diseases
Ohio State University
Columbus, Ohio

Erica F. Lawson, MD (Questions 48, 49)
Clinical Fellow
Pediatric Rheumatology Fellow
University of California, San Francisco
San Francisco, California

Kimberly C. Martin, DO (Questions 13, 14, 15, 16)
Children's National Medical Center
Department of Pediatric Infectious Disease
Washington, DC

Debra L. Palazzi, MD (Questions 43, 44)
Assistant Professor of Pediatrics
Associate Fellowship Director
Infectious Diseases Section
Baylor College of Medicine
Texas Children's Hospital
Houston, Texas

José R. Romero, MD, FAAP (Questions 13, 14, 15, 16)
Professor of Pediatrics
Horace C. Cabe Chair in Infectious Diseases
Director, Pediatric Infectious Diseases Section
Arkansas Children's Hospital/University of Arkansas for Medical Sciences
Director, Clinical Trials Research
Arkansas Children's Hospital Research Institute
Arkansas Children's Hospital
Little Rock, Arkansas

Masako Shimamura, MD (Questions 39, 40, 41, 42)
Associate Professor, Pediatric Infectious Diseases
Department of Pediatrics
University of Alabama at Birmingham
Birmingham, Alabama

Kevin B. Spicer, MD, PhD, MPH (Questions 23, 24, 25, 26, 27)
Assistant Professor, Department of Pediatrics
College of Medicine, The Ohio State University
Attending Physician, Section of Infectious Diseases
Nationwide Children's Hospital
Columbus, Ohio

Laura Patricia Stadler, MEd, MD, MS (Questions 45, 46)
Assistant Professor of Pediatrics
Pediatric Infectious Disease
Lexington, Kentucky

Emily A. Thorell, MD (Questions 5, 6, 7, 8)
Assistant Professor, Pediatric Infectious Disease
University of Utah
Director, Antimicrobial Stewardship Program
Associate Hospital Epidemiologist
Primary Children's Medical Center
Salt Lake City, Utah

Rene VanDeVoorde, MD (Questions 1, 2, 3, 4)
Assistant Professor, Pediatrics
Medical Director, Dialysis Unit
Cincinnati Children's Hospital
Cincinnati, Ohio

Rebecca W. Widener, MD (Questions 39, 40, 41, 42)
Pediatric Infectious Diseases Fellow
University of Alabama at Birmingham
Birmingham, Alabama

Preface

Much of the field of pediatric infectious disease centers on care of healthy children with acute infections. The infectious diseases highlighted in this book are commonly seen by the practicing pediatrician and family medicine physician. I created this book to address these common conditions with sometimes uncommon presentations. The clinical scenarios help to answer interesting questions that arise out of taking care of multitudes of patients, each of whom is slightly different from the next. Each question in this book helps to arm the clinician with clinical solutions for a range of diagnoses and supports a common-sense approach to more unusual and less common illnesses. To accomplish this goal, I was fortunate enough to have an expert group of pediatric clinicians from across several subspecialties to evaluate the most current literature and then write in a succinct format for the busy clinician. This book is also useful for nurse practitioners, physician assistants, medical students, and pediatric and family medicine residents for practical answers related to specific patients or as a learning tool for furthering education.

Foreword

Providing medical care for children carries considerable responsibility, as children are the seeds of our future. In providing that care, the best medical advice is based on scientific evidence from well-conducted clinical studies. The volume of new knowledge is rapidly expanding and can overwhelm the practicing physician. In addition, the growth of new sources of information, both original data and thoughtful and authoritative syntheses of original data, is exponential. Practice guidelines, expert panel reports, survey results, professional society recommendations, and review articles have proliferated both in the print media and on the Internet. At the same time, the routine practice of pediatric medicine has recently undergone considerable change, led by evolving financial considerations and constraints, the availability of new treatment modalities, changes in the organization of health care delivery, and increasing drug shortages that force new uses of alternative agents to treat ill children. As a result, physicians now have less time to wade through the exploding literature to answer the many patient care questions that emerge in their clinical practices.

The field of infectious diseases, a vibrant, ever-changing subspecialty in pediatrics, is also central to the practice of general pediatrics and crosses every medical and surgical pediatric discipline. Children get infections. Often. Some are more serious than others, but many require medical expertise for appropriate management. In addition, the consequences of treatment strategies for infections in children extend beyond the ill child, as the use of antibiotics plays a huge role in driving antibiotic resistance in bacteria colonizing the ill child and others in his or her community. Further, the financial costs of the management of infectious diseases in children are borne by our entire society.

Thus, *Curbside Consultation in Pediatric Infectious Disease: 49 Clinical Questions* has arrived at an ideal time to assist physicians who care for children. The format—referenced, thoughtful, informative answers to 49 clinical questions commonly encountered in pediatric practice—reflects the way physicians use medical knowledge. The value of the book includes the choice of pertinent questions, the experience of the authors, the inclusion of easy-to-access tables and figures, and the short, informative, to-the-point answers.

To the readers: treasure this important resource; enjoy access to the wisdom within its pages; use it in your practices. To the patients of the readers: you are fortunate, indeed.

Janet R. Gilsdorf, MD
Robert P. Kelch Research Professor
Director, Pediatric Infectious Diseases
University of Michigan Medical Center
Ann Arbor, Michigan

Introduction

We wrote this book for the busy clinician. It is appropriate for both specialists and primary care providers and is designed to be a ready guide for common clinical questions involving pediatric infections as well as illnesses that mimic common infections. The questions of this book are divided into categories including gastrointestinal, respiratory, immune system evaluation and dysfunction, diseases that mimic infection, skin/soft tissue, and lymph node infections. Common office topics such as recurrent otitis media and sinusitis are covered, as well as recurrent thrush, diarrhea, methicillin-resistant *Staphylococcus aureus*, and community-acquired pneumonia. Less common, but important to recognize issues include cat-scratch disease, Kawasaki syndrome, Epstein-Barr virus, cytomegalovirus, periodic fever syndromes, and immune system dysfunction, to name a few. The overarching goal of this book is to provide ready answers to some common and uncommon clinical scenarios. The contributors to this book are experts in their fields and have provided concise, but detailed information for the clinician on the go. It is our sincere hope that the reader enjoys this book as much as we enjoyed writing and putting the content together.

SECTION I

URINARY TRACT INFECTION

IS IT APPROPRIATE TO TREAT A SUSPECTED URINARY TRACT INFECTION BASED ON AN IN-OFFICE URINE DIPSTICK RESULT, OR SHOULD THE SPECIMEN BE SENT FOR CULTURE? DOES THE AGE OF THE PATIENT HAVE ANYTHING TO DO WITH THE DECISION?

Rene VanDeVoorde, MD

Urine culture remains the criterion standard for diagnosis of urinary tract infection (UTI). Urine is usually sterile and thus any bacteria growing in it should be considered an infection. However, children may have asymptomatic bacteriuria or contamination of the collected specimen such that bacteria may grow on culture without any symptoms being present. Early studies showed that adult patients often could have some bacteria growing in culture, but only after there was a certain concentration of bacteria would UTI symptoms also be present. Because of this threshold for causing symptoms and the variation in contamination rates by the urine collection method, there are different standards for what constitutes a positive urine culture (Table 1-1) of a single organism.

The biggest problem with a urine culture is the delay in receiving results, a minimum of 24 to 36 hours for most laboratories, with even longer waits for antibiotic susceptibilities. Also, depending on your medical practice, cultures may be incubated in the office, requiring appropriate equipment and personnel training, or elsewhere, with potentially even longer delays in receiving results. Therefore, there has been keen interest in the accuracy of more rapid urine testing, such as dipstick (leukocyte esterase [LE], nitrite) and microscopy (pyuria, bacteriuria), for predicting UTI.

The presence of bacteria on microscopy of an uncentrifuged urine specimen has been shown to be the single test with the highest specificity and sensitivity for UTI, as reported by 2 separate meta-analyses (Table 1-2).[1,2] The presence of pyuria (>5 white blood cells/high-powered field) on microscopic examination of a centrifuged specimen does not have as high a sensitivity or specificity as bacteriuria, but when the 2 are present together,

Table 1-1

Colony Counts of Single Organisms for Positive Urine Culture by Collection Method

Urine Collection Method	Colony, Counts/mL, of a Single Organism
Suprapubic aspiration	Any number, for gram-negative bacilli $>10^3$ (>1000) for gram-positive cocci
Urethral catheterization	$>10^4$ (>10,000) = infection likely $>10^5$ (>100,000) = positive
Clean voided	$>10^4$ (>10,000) in boys $>10^5$ (>100,000) in girls

Adapted from Downs SM. Practice parameter: the diagnosis, treatment, and evaluation of the initial urinary tract infection in febrile infants and young children. American Academy of Pediatrics. Committee on Quality Improvement. Subcommittee on Urinary Tract Infection. *Pediatrics.* 1999;103(4, pt 1):843-852.[1]

Table 1-2

Diagnostic Accuracy of Different Rapid Urine Testing for Urinary Tract Infection

Test	Sensitivity[1], %	Specificity[1], %	+LR[3]	−LR[3]
LE alone	84	77	5.5	0.26
Nitrite alone	58	99	15.9	0.51
LE or nitrite	92	70	6.1	0.2
LE + nitrite	–	–	28.2	0.37
Pyuria (>5 wbc)	78	87	5.9	0.27
Bacteriuria	88	93	14.7	0.19
Pyuria or bacteriuria	–	–	4.2	0.11
Pyuria + bacteriuria	–	–	37.0	0.21

LE = leukocyte esterase, +LR = positive likelihood ratio, −LR = negative likelihood ratio.

Adapted from Downs SM. Practice parameter: the diagnosis, treatment, and evaluation of the initial urinary tract infection in febrile infants and young children. American Academy of Pediatrics. Committee on Quality Improvement. Subcommittee on Urinary Tract Infection. *Pediatrics.* 1999;103(4, pt 1):843-852[1] and Whiting P, Westwood M, Watt I, et al. Rapid tests and urine sampling techniques for the diagnosis of urinary tract infection (UTI) in children under five years of age: a systematic review. *BMC Pediatr.* 2005;5:4.[3]

the likelihood of UTI is 2.5 times greater. The difficulties with microscopic examination of the urine are that it requires additional time for preparation of the specimen (Gram staining, centrifugation), involves equipment that is not readily available in most practice settings, and should be performed regularly to maintain diagnostic acumen.

Hence, urine dipstick is often the most utilized rapid test of urine. The presence of LE and nitrite has also been evaluated for their diagnostic accuracy, both individually and in combination (see Table 1-2). The presence of nitrites has great specificity for UTI and should be used to rule in infection. However, because the bacterial conversion of nitrate to nitrite is not inherent to many gram-positive cocci, such as *Enterococcus spp*, this test can yield a false-negative result in these cases and has a low sensitivity. Dipstick LE is often graduated from trace to 4+, which may explain its lower reported specificity in the literature. Hence, a "more positive" LE is likely more specific for the presence of true infection. The presence of both LE and nitrite has the highest positive likelihood ratio (LR) for a positive urine culture, whereas the absence of both has the lowest (best) negative LR in young (<5 years old) children.[3] However, a comparison of the diagnostic performance of urine dipstick in children younger than 2 years versus those 2 to 5 years old found that the LRs were significantly lower in the younger age group (7.62 versus 38.54 for positive LR, 0.34 versus 0.13 for negative LR).[4] Because both of these age groups have a high prevalence of UTI, especially in the scenario of a febrile female, these lower LRs may still be clinically relevant.

Many practitioners primarily rely upon urine dipstick results to steer decision making in patients who are not seriously ill. If both LE and nitrite are present on dipstick, it is reasonable to assume that a patient empirically has a UTI and treat as such. In a school-aged female (ie, able to verbalize symptoms appropriately) without pyelonephritis symptoms, a urine culture may be omitted with a convincingly positive urine dipstick, but it is important to make sure that she has a good clinical response to treatment within 48 hours. However, strong consideration should be given to sending a urine culture at the onset, in order to confirm the pathogen and appropriate antibiotic coverage, rather than waiting 48 hours for treatment failure before getting a culture. This is especially important in the era of rising antibiotic resistance. Additionally, knowledge of the local antibiogram is important when choosing an empiric therapy.

If a patient has a negative dipstick for both LE and nitrite, then a urine culture is not necessary unless the clinician feels the need to treat empirically. Those features that should prompt the clinician to treat empirically would include any ill or febrile infant younger than 60 days, a febrile infant with a previous history of UTI or urologic anomaly, or older children with pyelonephritis symptoms such as flank pain. In these cases, a negative culture at 48 hours can be used to help determine whether continuation of antibiotics is necessary or if further diagnostic testing (such as imaging) is necessary.

If a patient has a dipstick that is positive for only LE, then consideration should be given to sending a urine culture, with decision upon empiric treatment based on the patient's symptoms and clinical suspicion of UTI. Approaches similar to this have been published, such that if a dipstick (LE, nitrite) or microscopy (pyuria, bacteriuria) is positive for only one but not both tests, then cultures are required for determination.

Obtaining a urine culture is especially important in patients who are suspected of having or are known to have recurrent UTIs as these patients merit further evaluation (see Question 3). Therefore, it is important to first ensure that a patient is culture positive before embarking on any unnecessary and uncomfortable diagnostic testing.

Table 1-3

Other Diagnoses to Consider With Urinary Symptoms or Findings

Diagnoses	Similarities	Differentiating Findings
Dysfunctional voiding	Dysuria, enuresis, frequency	Urine withholding symptoms (peepee dance, Vincent's curtsy, grabbing)
Glomerulonephritis	Pyuria, gross hematuria, flank pain	Red cell casts, significant proteinuria, hypertension, edema
Kawasaki disease	Fever, pyuria	Cervical lymphadenopathy, rash, mucositis, digit swelling/peeling
Nephrolithiasis	Dysuria, flank pain, gross hematuria	Colicky pain, hypercalciuria, crystals on urine microscopy, stone on renal ultrasound or abdominal X-ray
Urethritis	Dysuria, pyuria	Urethral discharge, urine polymerase chain reaction for gonorrhea or chlamydia
Viral cystitis	Dysuria, gross hematuria, pyuria	Negative urine culture, adenovirus polymerase chain reaction
Vulvovaginitis or foreign body	Dysuria, pyuria	Perineal irritation, vaginal swab for Group A Strep, bloody or purulent discharge

There are several other disorders that may symptomatically masquerade like UTI (Table 1-3) and may only be differentiated by urine culture results. Often, UTI is presumptively diagnosed in the setting of gross hematuria, even in the absence of other UTI findings. In retrospect, these patients have either no culture obtained or a negative culture result. Therefore, it is recommended that a culture always be obtained as a part of this evaluation, unless the hematuria is clearly from another etiology.

Voiding dysfunction can be particularly difficult to diagnose and treat. These patients are often preschool– or early school–aged girls, a population with high prevalence for UTI. They often present with frequency, dysuria, or enuresis and have frequent symptomatic recurrences. Additionally, these patients are more susceptible to getting UTIs because of their poor bladder emptying. However, many of these patients do not have recurrent infections when cultured regularly. Therefore, consideration should be given to obtaining urine cultures consistently in these asymptomatic patients. Finally, in adolescents, sexually transmitted infections may mimic UTI with complaints of dysuria, whereas intercourse may also increase the risk of cystitis. It is also important to consider obtaining a urine culture, in addition to sexually transmitted infection testing, in these patients rather than providing empiric UTI treatment.

References

1. Downs SM. Practice parameter: the diagnosis, treatment, and evaluation of the initial urinary tract infection in febrile infants and young children. American Academy of Pediatrics. Committee on Quality Improvement. Subcommittee on Urinary Tract Infection. *Pediatrics.* 1999;103(4, pt 1):843-852.
2. Gorelick MH, Shaw KN. Screening tests for urinary tract infection in children: a meta-analysis. *Pediatrics.* 1999;104(5):e54.
3. Whiting P, Westwood M, Watt I, Cooper J, Kleijnen J. Rapid tests and urine sampling techniques for the diagnosis of urinary tract infection (UTI) in children under five years of age: a systematic review. *BMC Pediatr.* 2005;5:4.
4. Mori R, Yonemoto N, Fitzgerald A, Tullus K, Verrier-Jones K, Lakhanpaul L. Diagnostic performance of urine dipstick testing in children with suspected UTI: a systematic review of relationship with age and comparison with microscopy. *Acta Paediatr.* 2010;99(4):581-584.

WHEN SHOULD YOU ATTEMPT TO OBTAIN A CATHETER SPECIMEN VERSUS A CLEAN CATCH SPECIMEN IN THE SETTING OF A SUSPECTED URINARY TRACT INFECTION?

Rene VanDeVoorde, MD

For most children who are toilet trained, collecting a mid-stream clean catch specimen is perfectly apropos, given that proper technique is used for the collection. This approach has been supported in the adult literature showing that there is concordance of urinary test results for urinary tract infection (UTI) (culture, dipstick, and microscopy) between clean catch and catheterized urine specimens. However, as parents often may not accompany children into the restroom, one should have a low threshold of suspicion that proper collection technique is always being used, especially in younger patients. To appropriately obtain clean catch urine, the perineum should be cleansed with soap or an antiseptic solution prior to collection to reduce the risk of contamination. Antibacterial solution, such as povidine-iodine, should not be used as this could contaminate the specimen and cause false-negative culture results. For girls, the labia should be spread and the perineum cleansed 2 or 3 times. For boys, the meatus should be cleansed similarly, with uncircumcised boys retracting their foreskin to do so. Spreading the labia or retraction of the foreskin should be maintained while voiding to minimize mucosal contact with the urine stream. Midway through the void, a specimen should be collected into a sterile urine cup. This may be difficult for many adults to perform, so the clinician may need to emphasize the need for proper technique and potential parental assistance to obtain a specimen accurately.

There is 1 situation in which strong consideration should be given to obtaining a catheterized specimen in a stable patient who is otherwise toilet trained—the patient who is repeatedly having "contaminated" urine cultures (mixed flora, >3 organisms, or skin flora). In this instance, a catheterized specimen may help to confirm or deny suspicions of whether the patient is having genuine UTIs. If medical care is received from different

Table 2-1

Reported Risks of Catheterization

Risk	Frequency
Trauma	Microscopic hematuria (17%), stenosis
Substantial discomfort	6% during investigative studies
Infection	3% for investigative studies, lower for in-and-out catheterization
Catheter knotting	0.2/100,000 catheterizations
Inadequate specimen	4% (with bladder ultrasound), 23% to 28%

providers in different settings (after-hours clinic, emergency room), the pattern of recurrence may be missed. Also, *Staphylococcus epidermidis saprophyticus* are often thought of as skin contaminants, but they can be true uropathogens as well. Therefore, one should be wary to overlook a positive culture for either of these agents, especially if the culture had high colony counts (>10^5) or the patient has classic symptoms.

For children who are not toilet trained, which includes nearly all infants, this question becomes more difficult and weighs the needs of the clinician for accurate testing (and the consequences of inaccuracy) versus the patient's, and the family's need to minimize discomfort from any procedure. Suprapubic catheterization (aspiration) of the bladder is often reported as the "criterion standard" for accurate urine testing. However, it is the most "invasive," its success rate obtaining urine is low, and frankly it is not routinely performed by (or even taught to) many practitioners who have completed training in the last 10 years. Therefore, for practical purposes, the rest of the discussion henceforth focuses only on in-and-out urethral catheterization of the bladder. This procedure, though less invasive, is not without risks (Table 2-1), but these risks may be minimized by appropriate sizing and lubrication of the catheter, use of local anesthetics to the urethral opening, appropriate discussion with parents, and skill of the performing provider.

Less-invasive methods to collect urine typically include the use of an adhesive bag placed over the perineum, cotton balls or pads placed in the diaper, or direct collection from the diaper itself. Obtaining a urine specimen by using cotton balls or directly sampling from diapers is not a clean catch per se and has a high risk of contamination, although data are not necessarily conclusive that these methods are any worse. However, for cleanly "caught" bag urine, the urine bag should directly adhere to the patient's skin, be changed every 30 minutes, and be removed shortly after the patient has voided to minimize contamination.

There are 2 patients for which the clinician should never rely upon a clean catch specimen for the diagnosis of UTI—infants younger than 90 days or ill-appearing children—as the stakes are too great with a missed diagnosis. In both situations, it is prudent to accurately obtain a urine culture, which should never be done from a "bagged" specimen. Therefore, a catheterized specimen would need to be obtained anyway. A study in infants comparing the culture results collected in these 2 ways yielded a contamination rate of nearly 63% with

Table 2-2
Comparison of Sensitivity and Specificity of Bag Versus Catheter Urine Specimens

Test/Statistic	Bag	Catheter	P
Dipstick/sensitivity	0.85	0.71	0.003
Microscopy/sensitivity	0.95	0.83	0.004
Dipstick/specificity	0.62	0.97	<0.001
Microscopy/specificity	0.45	0.95	<0.001

Adapted from McGillivray D, Mok E, Mulrooney E, et al. A head-to-head comparison: "clean-void" bag versus catheter urinalysis in the diagnosis of urinary tract infection in young children. *J Pediatr.* 2005;147(4):451-456.[2]

bag samples (versus 9% by catheter) and increased odds of unnecessary treatment, radiologic evaluation, and hospital admission. A separate study showed that 40% of cultures from bag specimens led to a misdiagnosis, compared to only 5.7% in catheterized specimens.[1]

However, in infants who are at low risk for UTI, urinalysis results from a cleanly voided "bagged" specimen may be useful. The sensitivity of a "bagged" specimen is greater for both urine dipstick and microscopy than catheterized urine specimens (Table 2-2),[2] although it has lower specificity. Therefore, "bagged" urine whose results are negative for both leukocyte esterase and nitrite on dipstick (or pyuria and bacteria on microscopy) can be useful for ruling out UTI and the need for confirmatory culture. However, if either test gives a positive result, then a culture is needed and this should only be obtained by catheterization.

So, if an infant patient has a low risk for UTI (no previous history of UTI, no known urologic abnormalities, no fever, not ill-appearing, >90 days old, circumcised), it is reasonable to consider first obtaining a bagged urine specimen and, if negative, avoid the need for catheterization. However, if there is high suspicion that a urine culture will be needed anyway, such as an evaluation for fever, it is prudent to obtain a catheterized specimen from the onset.

References

1. Etoubleau C, Reveret M, Brouet D, et al. Moving from bag to catheter for urine collection in non-toilet-trained children suspected of having urinary tract infection: a paired comparison of urine cultures. *J Pediatr.* 2009;154(6):803-806.
2. McGillivray D, Mok E, Mulrooney E, Kramer MS. A head-to-head comparison: "clean-void" bag versus catheter urinalysis in the diagnosis of urinary tract infection in young children. *J Pediatr.* 2005;147(4):451-456.

Suggested Reading

Wald ER. To bag or not to bag. *J Pediatr.* 2005;147(4):418-420.

WHEN IS IMAGING, SUCH AS VOIDING CYSTOURETHROGRAM AND RENAL ULTRASOUND, NECESSARY FOR CHILDREN WITH A FIRST URINARY TRACT INFECTION?

Rene VanDeVoorde, MD

The goal of radiologic imaging of the genitourinary tract with urinary tract infection (UTI) for many is to answer the question of whether a patient is more predisposed to long-term adverse effects from infections. A patient may be considered low risk for adverse effects if he or she is toilet-trained; presents with only his or her first (or second) UTI; presents only with symptoms that are isolated to the lower urinary tract such as frequency, urgency, and dysuria; and has a negative family history for significant renal or urologic disorders. So if a school-aged female presented with dysuria and was found to have her first UTI, pursuit of any radiologic imaging at that time is not obligatory. However, patients who could potentially have pyelonephritis (younger than 3 years; febrile, flank pain, ill appearance; or family history of high-grade reflux), are not typical for developing cystitis (males, especially if circumcised), or have recurrent infections merit at least an initial evaluation.

Many have inferred that this evaluation is simply to document the presence of high-grade vesicoureteral reflux (VUR) and, hence, the risk of recurrent pyelonephritis and renal scarring. However, the purpose of this evaluation may not only be to rule out the risk of recurrent pyelonephritis but also to assuage parental, and clinician, fears of other significant abnormalities of the genitourinary tract. Thus, the focus should also include consideration of other pathologies, not restricted just to VUR, for which a UTI could simply be the initial presentation.

Because a renal ultrasound (US) is noninvasive and evaluates the urinary collecting system for dilation as well as the morphology, size, and echogenicity of the kidneys, it gives a facile, cursory look for any frank anatomical anomalies and can be used to give some reassurance to families that there is not a significant problem with their child's urinary tract. Some studies in the literature contend that renal US has a low yield for

Table 3-1

Renal Ultrasound Findings Associated With Increased Risk of or Complications From Urinary Tract Infection

Acute pyelonephritis or renal scarring
Renal hypoplasia or dysplasia
Hydronephrosis, hydroureter, or dilation of the pelvicaliceal system
Bladder wall thickening
Bladder diverticula or trabeculation*
Horseshoe kidney
Ectopic kidney
Solitary kidney*
Duplex collecting system
Renal calculus

*Adapted from Lee MD, Lin CC, Huang FY, et al. Screening young children with a first febrile urinary tract infection for high-grade vesicoureteral reflux with renal ultrasound scanning and technetium-99m-labeled dimercaptosuccinic acid scanning. *J Pediatr.* 2009;154(6):797-802.[1]

predicting VUR or the presence of pyelonephritis and should not be considered in the initial evaluation. However, in a retrospective study of infants and toddlers with their first febrile UTI, renal US uncovered abnormalities (Table 3-1) in 56% of all patients and had a negative predictive value for reflux of 87%.[1] US may also give supplemental information about a child's risk for lower tract infections by showing bladder abnormalities, which may not be as easily revealed by other radiographic studies. For these aforementioned reasons, a renal US should not be passed over and ought to be the initially ordered study.

Some endorse that a renal US is not indicated with a first febrile UTI if there was a normal prenatal US performed after 30 to 32 weeks gestation by an experienced obstetrical center. However, this is not a frequently performed test in most pregnancies. When it has been done, access to the radiologist report (to confirm a normal result) or the ability to reliably interpret prenatal imaging (as one would do for postnatal imaging) is lacking. Thus, acceptable prenatal imaging, or the ability to sufficiently review it, when it has been obtained, often does not exist.

Obtaining a voiding cystourethrogram (VCUG) with first UTI in all male patients, females younger than 3 years (often by default those who are not toilet trained), children clinically suspected of having pyelonephritis (fever >101, flank pain), and those with US abnormalities has been recommended.[2] This is important, as VCUG is the only way to assuredly evaluate for the presence of VUR, and prophylactic antibiotics are still indicated in cases of high-grade reflux (see Question 4). However, if it is later shown that there is no benefit from antibiotic prophylaxis in patients with higher grades (III–V) of reflux,

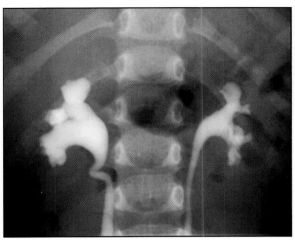

Figure 3-1. Bilateral vesicoureteral reflux. VCUG showing Grade 4 reflux on the right (severe blunting of the calyces, pelvic dilation, and ureteral tortuosity) and Grade 3 reflux on the left (some blunting of the calyces). (Reprinted with permission of Steven Kraus, MD, Cincinnati Children's Hospital Medical Center.)

then this approach should be reconsidered. Additionally, it is important to talk frankly with families about the diagnostic and therapeutic approach to VUR. If the family is disinclined to use prophylaxis in the case of higher grade VUR (Figure 3-1), understands the risks, and acknowledges the need for prompt evaluation when their child is febrile, then it is reasonable to pursue a VCUG only if there are changes on US.

Also, the VCUG may be obtained soon after diagnosis, including during an inpatient hospitalization, as long as the patient has clinically responded to treatment. Previously it was thought that a delay after infection was needed for a VCUG to have diagnostic validity, because the bladder inflammation from an acute UTI would increase the likelihood of seeing reflux and give more false-positive results. However, this is not the case. Further, it is more likely that an ordered VCUG will not be completed if there is a delay of a few weeks in scheduling it after infection. Additionally, there is a small chance of introducing bacteria into the urinary tract, thus causing UTI during a VCUG, which would not be of concern if the patient is still receiving his or her treatment course of antibiotics at the time of the study's performance.

Because of the risks and cost of the VCUG test, as well as its low yield (<10%) for clinically significant (ie, high-grade) VUR, many have advocated obtaining VCUGs selectively. The National Institute for Health and Clinical Excellence (NICE) in the United Kingdom has published guidelines for the approach to UTI in children,[3] recommending routine VCUG only in infants younger than 6 months who have a recurrence or atypical feature (seriously ill including fever >39°C, non-*Escherichia coli* organisms, poor urine flow, palpable abdominal mass, elevated creatinine, septicemia, or poor response in 48 hours) to their UTI. Their only considerations for obtaining a VCUG in older infants and toddlers are those who have dilation on US findings, poor urine flow, or family histories of high-grade VUR. Studies have shown that these guidelines can miss a substantial number of patients with reflux or scarring, although it is unclear how clinically significant these omissions are long term.

Another approach to imaging is the so-called "top-down" approach, where renal scintigraphy, or dimercaptosuccinic acid (DMSA) scan is obtained initially, with other studies contingent on the scintigraphic findings. Advocates of this approach cite that it focuses on identification of renal scarring, the long-term adverse effect that we are hoping to

Figure 3-2. Acute pyelonephritis on renal scintigraphy. DMSA scan with views highlighting each kidney individually. Pyelonephritis or renal scarring is present in 2 areas of the left kidney, represented by hypodense, or lucent, areas of the lower pole and the medial upper pole. (Reprinted with permission of Steven Kraus, MD, Cincinnati Children's Hospital Medical Center.)

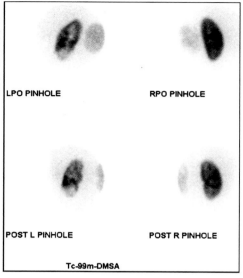

avoid, regardless of whether reflux is present.[4] DMSA scans performed acutely have high specificity for acute pyelonephritis (Figure 3-2), so they may be used as a screening tool for those at risk for having significant VUR leading to pyelonephritis. Studies have cited high negative predictive values for higher grades of VUR with normal DMSA scans and the possibility of avoiding unnecessary VCUGs. However, negative DMSA scans do not conclusively rule out all cases of higher grade reflux and are associated with higher doses of gonadal radiation exposure. Positive DMSA results in the acute setting of pyelonephritis do not always correlate to renal scarring, with as few as 15% of acute findings leading to permanent scarring, so that an additional scan performed 3 to 6 months later is needed to confirm the presence of permanent scarring. Finally, as this test has not traditionally been used, both its availability outside of the academic setting and the radiologist's comfort level in performing it should be confirmed before pursuing it as a standard diagnostic tool.

References

1. Lee MD, Lin CC, Huang FY, Tsai TC, Huang CT, Tsai JD. Screening young children with a first febrile urinary tract infection for high-grade vesicoureteral reflux with renal ultrasound scanning and technetium-99m-labeled dimercaptosuccinic acid scanning. *J Pediatr.* 2009;154(6):797-802.
2. Cincinnati Children's Hospital Medical Center. Evidence-based care guideline for medical management of first urinary tract infection in children 12 years of age or less. http://www.cincinnatichildrens.org/svc/alpha/h/health-policy/uti.htm. Accessed November 1, 2010.
3. National Institute for Health and Clinical Excellence. NICE Guideline 54—Urinary tract infection: diagnosis, treatment and long-term management of urinary tract infection in children. http://www.nice.org.uk/nicemedia/pdf/CG54algorithm.pdf
4. Pohl HG, Belman AB. The "top-down" approach to the evaluation of children with febrile urinary tract infection. *Adv Urol.* 2009;2009:783-409.

IS PROPHYLAXIS RECOMMENDED FOR ALL PATIENTS WITH VESICOURETERAL REFLUX?

Rene VanDeVoorde, MD

The association of urinary tract infection (UTI) and vesicoureteral reflux (VUR) with renal damage was made more than 40 years ago and led to the recommended practice of assessing for VUR in children who had UTIs. Similarly, it was thought that the prevention of UTI by daily administration of low-dose antibiotics would lead to decreased renal injury in patients with VUR, as animal models of reflux showed that subsequent episodes of infection, not just VUR, were needed for renal injury to occur. So, for over a decade, recommendations from organizations representing both urologists and pediatricians have supported giving antibiotics with most, if not all, grades of VUR. Recent studies have rightfully questioned the dogma that antibiotic prophylaxis benefits patients with VUR, raising skepticism of both their medical efficacy and cost-effectiveness. This has led to changes in practice by many pediatricians and subspecialists. However, it is important to note that not all of these studies are generally applicable to all patients with VUR because of their retrospective nature, differing patient populations (majority uncircumcised males, older patients, not all with VUR or lowest grades of VUR), or inadequate powering.

In addition to questioning the benefit of prophylactic antibiotics, there is growing concern of the potential harm from daily antibiotic exposure. Although given in lower doses than for treatment (Table 4-1), adverse effects can be seen. Additionally, in this era of increasing antimicrobial resistance, fear of indiscriminate antibiotic use is substantiated. A retrospective review of a large cohort of children with first UTI in the United States found that antibiotic prophylaxis did not decrease the risk of UTI recurring in patients with VUR but, in fact, was associated with an increased risk of subsequent UTI by resistant organisms.[1] A common approach, like that endorsed by these study authors, is to discuss the risks and potentially unclear benefits of prophylaxis with each family.

There are 2 groups of VUR patients in whom the approach has remained largely unchanged over the years, those with the highest (5) and lowest (1) grades. In patients with Grade 5 VUR, antibiotic prophylaxis should be instituted and only allowed to be discontinued after discussions with the consulting urologist. Often this degree of reflux

Table 4-1

Recommended Dosing of Different Antibiotics for Urinary Tract Infection Prophylaxis

Drug Name	Daily Dosing	Comments/Potential Adverse Reactions
Amoxicillin	10 mg/kg	Increased resistance is noted
Cefixime	4 mg/kg	High cost, difficult to find
Cephalexin	10 mg/kg	Liquid form may only be good for 14 days
Ciprofloxacin	1 mg/kg	Broad spectrum; not used in younger children
Nitrofurantoin	1 to 2 mg/kg	Bone marrow suppression; bad taste; not used in newborn period
Sulfamethoxazole/trimethoprim (TMP)	2 mg/kg of TMP	Stevens-Johnson syndrome; bone marrow suppression; not in newborn period (jaundice)

is already associated with some degree of renal injury, such that one should be wary of risking any further loss of functional tissue. This feeling is likely shared by many others as this population has been excluded from nearly every recent randomized control trial involving interventions, including the ongoing Randomized Intervention for Children with Vesicoureteral Reflux (RIVUR) study.[2]

In patients with Grade 1 VUR, prophylactic antibiotics are generally not recommended for the prevention of pyelonephritis episodes. This conflicts with the original recommendations of the American Urological Association, which endorsed treating all grades of reflux. As Grade I VUR does not reach the level of the kidney (Figure 4-1), it should pose little risk of directly causing pyelonephritis and renal scarring. So, antibiotic prophylaxis is not recommended, and consideration should be given to talking parents out of prophylaxis in this instance.

In patients with VUR of Grades 2 to 4, the approach should be tailored to the clinical situation and family desires after frank discussion of the risks and benefits of both prophylaxis and no prophylaxis. For patients with Grade 2 VUR, discussion should include the fact that the reflux is up to the level of the kidney so that, in theory, infected urine could ascend to the kidney while tempering this with the facts that most cases of Grade 2 VUR resolve with time and more recent studies have shown little association with kidney scarring. With Grade 3 VUR, there is decreased likelihood of resolution, which should be explained to the family. However, there is also a lack of association with kidney scarring. It is important to note that antibiotic prophylaxis has been associated with a reduction in UTIs with Grade 3 VUR,[3] albeit only in boys. With Grade 4 VUR, it is important to highlight that the reflux is unlikely to completely resolve, although it may decrease in severity with time, and has been associated with an increased risk of UTI recurrence.[1] Also, Grade 4 VUR has been associated with worsening renal function on

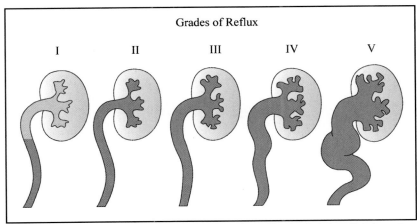

Figure 4-1. Grading of vesicoureteral reflux. Grade I—into distal ureter, Grade II—up into renal pelvis and calyces without dilation, Grade III—with mild dilation of pelvis and calyces, Grade IV—with moderate dilation of ureter and pelvis and moderate blunting of the calyces, Grade V—gross dilation and tortuosity of the ureter and pelvis and significant blunting of the calyces. (Adapted from Evidence-Based Care Guideline for Medical Management of First Urinary Tract Infection in Children, Cincinnati Children's Hospital Medical Center.)

follow-up dimercaptosuccinic acid (DMSA) scans, although not always due to recurring infections. This last fact highlights clinicians' concerns that patients with higher grades of reflux are at greater risk due to the potential of less functional renal parenchyma at baseline.

When pressed by parents asking the sometimes dreaded, "What would you do if this was your child?" I share that I would not, as a rule, start prophylaxis with Grade 2, but would in Grades 3 and 4 VUR. However, I also share that this view has evolved over time and may change again. The ongoing RIVUR study in the United States hopes to answer many of the questions regarding prophylaxis and reflux, as it seems to address many of the flaws of earlier studies with its prospective nature, adequate sample size (>500), inclusion only of patients with VUR, and use of placebo.[2]

Even if studies conclusively find a benefit to antibiotic prophylaxis in VUR, there is still another question to be answered about their use: "How long should prophylaxis be administered?" The correct answer is until the patient's risk has resolved, but what is truly placing the patient at risk is often more difficult to determine. For many practitioners, their answer may be simple—until the reflux is resolved or becomes low grade, but this requires periodic checking by repeat voiding cystourethrogram (VCUG). For other patients, their biggest risk factor may be their lack of toilet-training or their inability to verbalize early symptoms. In each instance, conversations, including specific scenarios such as these, with families should be pursued so that they can be part of the decision-making process of developing criteria for discontinuation of prophylaxis. In general, patients who are started on prophylaxis should be maintained for a minimum of 6 months without significant breakthrough infections.

Finally, use of antibiotic prophylaxis is not limited only to patients with VUR. In patients who have frequently recurring cystitis without reflux, a short course of antibiotic prophylaxis is reasonable. The intention is to break the recurring cycle of lower tract infection, which may lead to poor bladder emptying, and an increased risk of infection. This approach is supported by the findings of the Australian PRIVENT study, which found that antibiotic prophylaxis prevented UTI and febrile UTI recurrence in children when compared with placebo, irrespective of their VUR status.[4] An optimal time period for prophylaxis in these instances has not been determined, but a similar period of 6 months seems a reasonable approach. Incidentally, this was the same period that was found to have the greatest reduction in infections in this study. The period of prophylaxis is an ideal time for the family to work on appropriate bladder hygiene and address contributing factors to dysfunctional voiding, such as constipation and urine withholding, which have also been associated with recurrent UTIs.

References

1. Conway PH, Cnaan A, Zaoutis T, Henry BV, Grundmeier RW, Keren R. Recurrent urinary tract infections in children: risk factors and association with prophylactic antimicrobials. *JAMA*. 2007;298(2):179-186.
2. Keren R, Carpenter, MA, Hoberman A, et al. Rationale and design issues of the Randomized Intervention for Children with Vesicoureteral Reflux (RIVUR) study. *Pediatrics*. 2008;122(suppl 5):S240-S250.
3. Roussey-Kesler G, Gadjos V, Idres N, et al. Antibiotic prophylaxis for the prevention of recurrent urinary tract infection in children with low grade vesicoureteral reflux: results from a prospective randomized study. *J Urol*. 2008;179(2):674-679.
4. Craig JC, Simpson JM, Williams GJ, et al. Antibiotic prophylaxis and recurrent urinary tract infection in children. *N Engl J Med*. 2009;361(18):1748-1759.

SECTION II

METHICILLIN-RESISTANT
STAPHYLOCOCCUS AUREUS

WHEN IS ORAL ANTIBIOTIC THERAPY NECESSARY IN THE SETTING OF RECURRENT METHICILLIN-RESISTANT STAPHYLOCOCCUS AUREUS SKIN INFECTION/BOILS?

Emily A. Thorell, MD

It is unclear whether community-associated methicillin-resistant *Staphylococcus aureus* (MRSA) (CA-MRSA) skin and soft tissue infections (SSTIs) need to be treated differently from their methicillin-susceptible *S aureus* (MSSA) counterparts. We do know that both visits to emergency rooms and hospitalizations have increased for SSTI since the emergence of CA-MRSA. Studies of SSTI prior to this emergence showed that incision and drainage alone was adequate therapy for common purulent skin infections such as boils or furuncles. A nice randomized, double-blinded, placebo-controlled study in 50 adult patients in 1985 showed that antimicrobial therapy plus incision and drainage versus incision and drainage alone did not alter the patient's outcome after 1 week. In both groups, 96% of patients improved. Other studies have verified this finding.

This led investigators to wonder whether antimicrobial treatment is necessary for the treatment of CA-MRSA SSTI. There has certainly been concern that the emerging CA-MRSA may have different virulence factors and therefore may necessitate antimicrobial therapy. It is clear that incision and drainage will hasten recovery for those infections that have progressed to abscess, although some will drain on their own without a surgical procedure. In adults, a 2007 study randomized 166 outpatients with uncomplicated SSTI to placebo or cephalexin (first-generation cephalosporin) after incision and drainage. Despite 88% of the staphylococcal isolates being resistant to cephalexin, cure rates were 90% in the placebo arm and 84% in the cephalexin arm. In a pediatric study by Lee in 2004, incision and drainage without proper antibiotic therapy was found to be effective in the management of abscesses with a diameter less than 5 cm in immunocompetent children. This study also revealed that lesions more than 5 cm were a risk factor for hospitalization, but ineffective antimicrobial therapy did not increase risk for hospitalization.

Therefore, we can conclude that incision and drainage without antibiotics should be adequate for smaller CA-MRSA abscesses in healthy adults as well as in children. Unfortunately, there have been no clinical trials that evaluate the benefit of oral anti-microbials in the treatment of recurrent MRSA SSTI, in adults or children. Cases that would warrant empiric antibiotic therapy would be those patients who are at risk to have progressive disseminated infection. These include patients who are immu-nocompromised or with other comorbidities, infants and the elderly, anyone with signs or symptoms of systemic illness, and those with associated thrombophlebitis. Hospitalization and intravenous therapy may also be required depending on the severity. Patients who have failed incision and drainage or those in whom incision and drainage is difficult based on location of the infection (eg, genitalia) are likely to benefit from antimicrobial therapy as well.

Choosing the right antibiotic in this era of CA-MRSA is much more challenging than in the past. There are also many patients who present for care of a SSTI when empiric anti-biotic therapy is often prescribed without an identifiable organism, so we have to make our best guess. Patients with simple, superficial skin infections such as impetigo may respond solely to topical therapy with mupirocin. Traditionally, the beta-lactam agents (ie, cephalexin or amoxicillin/clavulanate), which are active against both *S aureus* and Group A streptococcus (GAS), have been the first-line oral therapy. These agents are not active against CA-MRSA; therefore, oral antibiotic options are more limited. In children, the mainstays include clindamycin and trimethoprim-sulfamethoxazole (TMP/SMX). Tetracyclines (doxycycline or minocycline) and linezolid are also options; however, tooth staining in children younger than 8 with tetracyclines and the prohibitive cost of linezolid make these options less desirable. Clindamycin may also be difficult to prescribe for young children who cannot swallow pills as the unpleasant taste of the liquid solution is infamous, and limited concentrations are available, making dosing difficult in the bigger child. However, capsule formulation may be an alternative for the older child who cannot swallow a pill, as it can be opened and sprinkled on food.

It is important to remember that TMP/SMX and tetracyclines are not active against GAS. If coverage for GAS, MSSA, and CA-MRSA is desired, clindamycin or linezolid alone or combinations of a beta-lactam along with TMP/SMX or a tetracycline are neces-sary. The addition of rifampin as an adjunctive therapy is recommended by some experts when treating CA-MRSA disease, but rifampin should never be used alone as resistance emerges rapidly. Vancomycin is generally the first-line intravenous agent when CA-MRSA is suspected in a systemically ill child. Figure 5-1 illustrates an algorithm from the Centers for Disease Control and Prevention (CDC) for initial management of SSTIs.

It is important to know what the local epidemiology of *S aureus* is in the community prior to making antibiotic decisions. The list of susceptibilities (antibiogram) for organ-isms from the local hospitals should be available to aid in decision making. If the staphy-lococcal isolate is methicillin resistant, the susceptibility report will list it as oxacillin or nafcillin resistant as methicillin is not used clinically. Clindamycin resistance is emerging but rates vary widely in different communities. There is an interesting phenomenon with clindamycin as the bacteria may carry a gene (erythromycin ribosomal methylase or *erm*) that can induce clindamycin resistance. The phenotypic marker of this is a standard sus-ceptibility report that shows the organism as resistant to erythromycin but susceptible to

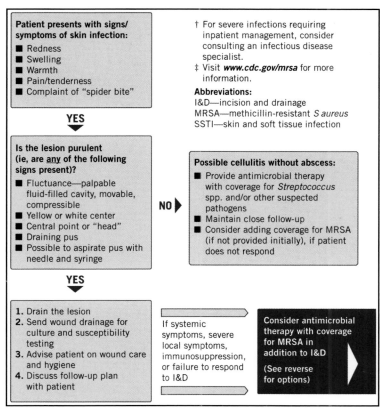

Figure 5-1. Algorithm guiding the outpatient management of CA-MRSA skin and soft tissue infections. (Reprinted with permission of the Centers for Disease Control and Prevention. MRSA; 2010. www.cdc.gov/mrsa/treatment/outpatient-management.html.)

clindamycin. Since 2004, all laboratories should be performing an additional test called the D-test on isolates with this phenotypic pattern to look for this inducible resistance. If the D-test is positive, clinicians should be aware that treatment failures with clindamycin are likely with repeated or extended use.

In those patients for whom drainage is possible, a culture of the abscess fluid or pustule is generally warranted in the era of CA-MRSA. Although a drainage procedure may be curative in and of itself, if treatment failure occurs, culture will reveal the organism as well as susceptibility to determine appropriate antibiotic therapy. It is also useful to monitor for changes in susceptibility patterns for those with recurrent disease.

Suggested Readings

Lee MC, Rios AM, Aten MF, et al. Management and outcome of children with skin and soft tissue abscesses caused by methicillin-resistant *Staphylococcus aureus*. Pediatr Infect Dis J. 2004;23(2):123-127.

Liu C, Bayer A, Cosgrove SE et al. Clinical practice guidelines by the Infectious Diseases Society of America for the treatment of methicillin-resistant *Staphylococcus aureus* Infection in adults and children. *Clin Infect Dis.* 2011; 52(3):e18-e55.

Llera JL, Levy RC. Treatment of cutaneous abscess: a double-blind clinical study. *Ann Emerg Med.* 1985;14(1):15-19.

Rajendran PM, Young D, Maurer T, et al. Randomized, double-blind, placebo-controlled trial of cephalexin for treatment of uncomplicated skin abscesses in a population at risk for community-acquired methicillin-resistant *Staphylococcus aureus* infection. *Antimicrob Agents Chemother.* 2007;51(11):4044-4048.

ARE BLEACH BATHS OR CHLORHEXIDINE PLUS MUPIROCIN OINTMENT USEFUL TO DECOLONIZE PATIENTS WITH RECURRENT METHICILLIN-RESISTANT STAPHYLOCOCCUS AUREUS INFECTIONS? WHAT TOPICAL RECOMMENDATIONS ARE USEFUL FOR PATIENTS WITH RECURRENT INFECTIONS?

Emily A. Thorell, MD

Recurrent community-associated MRSA (CA-MRSA) infections have become a tremendous burden for practitioners, patients, and their families. Many experts recommend decolonization protocols for patients with recurrent MRSA skin and soft tissue infections (SSTIs) as an attempt to decrease this burden. It is unclear from the literature whether decolonization with bleach or chlorhexidine plus or minus mupirocin ointment to colonized areas really works for recurrent MRSA. In addition, the optimal strategy to reduce or eradicate MRSA and prevent recurrence in healthy children is unknown. The body of evidence is expanding but not definitive. Basic hygiene measures should always be used whether or not decolonization is attempted. These measures are expanded upon in Questions 7 and 8. It is also unclear how often these strategies should be employed if in fact they work at all. Let's look at the literature.

Recently, a randomized, investigator-blinded, placebo-controlled study looked at 31 patients with moderate-to-severe atopic dermatitis (eczema) with clinical signs of secondary bacterial infection. They were randomized to receive either nasal mupirocin and bleach baths (treatment) or nasal petrolatum and plain water baths (placebo) for 3 months. Interestingly, the study found that patients with eczema were less frequently colonized with MRSA than other pediatric patients in this hospital. Although 87% of the patients with eczema were colonized with SA from skin lesions, only 7.4% were noted to be MRSA; and

Figure 6-1. (A) Dose–response killing of control *S aureus* with increasing concentrations of hypochlorite incubated for 10 minutes at 37°C. Mean colony counts (CFU) of remaining live bacteria on logarithmic scale (n 4, SD). (B) Time course for the response of control *S aureus* for increasing incubation times, 2.5 µL/mL hypochlorite solutions incubated at 37°C Average colony counts of remaining live bacteria on logarithmic scale (n 5, SD). (Reproduced with permission of *Pediatric Inf Dis*, Vol. 27, Page 934, Copyright © 2008 by Wolters Kluwer.)

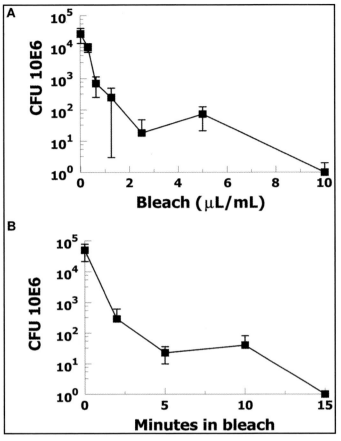

although 80% were colonized with SA in their nares, MRSA accounted for only 4%. During that time frame, MRSA was noted in 75% to 85% of SA cultures within the general population of this children's hospital. The good news was that the patients who were treated did have reduced severity of their atopic dermatitis. From this study, we can conclude that using mupirocin nasally along with bleach baths will help eczema patients who are infected with SA.

Another study looked at whether hypochlorite (bleach) actually kills MRSA to determine the optimal concentration and duration. It was determined that a concentration of 2.5 µL/mL dilution of bleach reduced the concentration of MRSA by 3 logs. Although higher doses achieved greater reduction in bacteria, the authors chose this dose as clinical experience suggested it was well tolerated by children. The authors then took this same concentration and measured the killing of bacteria over time. This showed that there was a 3 log decrease in the bacteria at 5 minutes, but a greater than 4 log decrease over 15 minutes (Figure 6-1). The 2.5-µL/mL dilution is equivalent to ½ cup (120 mL) of bleach in one-quarter filled standard tub (about 13 gallons). This is an in vitro study; therefore, it does not directly translate into decreasing the recurrence rate of MRSA SSTI. This concentration of bleach used on the skin of infected or colonized patients may help to decrease colonization and perhaps decrease recurrence, but this still needs further study in a clinical trial.

Chlorhexidine washes are also recommended by many experts. These are generally preferred by adults and older children who would rather use a shower than a bath. Most of the literature examining chlorhexidine is for both infection control in hospitals and prevention of catheter-associated and surgical site infections in both adults and children. For infection prevention purposes, chlorhexidine is becoming the preferred agent for sterile dressing changes and many surgical scrubs. Data as to whether this is also a good agent to address recurrent CA-MRSA SSTI are not available.

Mupirocin alone may be effective in reducing MRSA colonization, but it has not been shown to be sustained or to prevent recurrent infections among carriers. Reviews have shown that it may be useful in decreasing colonization in surgical and dialysis patients and reducing nosocomial infections in this population, but does not benefit nonsurgical patients. It has been used in adjunct to bleach or chlorhexidine by many experts. Using it in the nares alone may not be adequate as some patients are colonized in multiple or other areas. Conversely, the use of chlorhexidine wipes alone without nasal mupirocin does not appear to be effective.

Does the site of colonization matter? Approximately 25% to 30% of people are carriers of SA. In children, MRSA colonization rates have been reported anywhere from 0% to 22% depending on the location. Most of the focus of decolonization protocols has historically been the anterior nares, but other sites may be more likely to carry the bacteria. Sites of carriage include the anterior nares, perirectal area or perineum, and skin in general. Medical instrumentation such as tympanostomy tubes, gastrostomy tubes, tracheostomy tubes, and central lines can also be colonized. Another interesting study cultured the nares and rectum of 60 children with SA skin or soft tissue infection as well as 90 children without infection for control subjects. Sixty percent of the cases were MRSA and 40% MSSA. They found that SA was detected significantly more often in the rectum of children with abscesses (47%) than in the controls (1%). Nasal colonization was similar in both groups. Another interesting finding was that 88% of the SA recovered from the rectum was identical to the abscess culture. From this study, it seems that rectal colonization is actually a more important predictor of SSTI than nasal colonization, which may not be related at all.

Unfortunately, there are not good consensus guidelines regarding the use of mupirocin with or without bleach or chlorhexidine, so we rely on clinical experience and expert opinion. Most clinicians who see patients for recurrent MRSA infections will employ some of these techniques to try to help their patients when there is recurrent infection or transmission to other family members despite maximizing hygiene. It is common to try decolonization for all the members of a household when there is one member with recurrent disease as asymptomatic carriage is common as well. Hopefully, in the near future, we will have better guidance from the literature to help us make more evidence-based decisions for our patients.

Suggested Readings

Faden H, Lesse AJ, Trask J, et al. Importance of colonization site in the current epidemic of staphylococcal skin abscesses. *Pediatrics.* 2010;125(3):e618-e624.

Fisher RG, Chain RL, Hair PS, Cunnion KM. Hypochlorite killing of community-associated methicillin-resistant *Staphylococcus aureus. Pediatr Infect Dis J.* 2008;27(10):934-935.

Huang JT, Abrams M, Tlougan B, Rademaker A, Paller AS. Treatment of *Staphylococcus aureus* colonization in atopic dermatitis decreases disease severity. *Pediatrics.* 2009;123(5):e808-e814.

IN WHAT SETTINGS IS METHICILLIN-RESISTANT STAPHYLOCOCCUS AUREUS SPREAD?

Emily A. Thorell, MD

In thinking about how methicillin-resistant *Staphylococcus aureus* (MRSA) is spread, we need to look at the epidemiology of *Staphylococcus aureus* (SA). SA was discovered in Scotland in 1880 by a surgeon, Sir Alexander Ogston, from the drainage of a surgical abscess. He subsequently described its relation to suppurative inflammation as well as more invasive disease. Sadly, more than 130 years later and despite medical advances that Dr. Ogston could have never foreseen, we are still plagued by the same consequences of SA disease. SA is a ubiquitous organism; 25% to 30% of people are nasal carriers. The emergence of community-associated MRSA has changed the way clinicians think about how to prevent and treat *Staph aureus* infections, although it is far less ubiquitous. About 2% of people are colonized with MRSA, although this rate varies among different communities.

MRSA was first described in 1960 as a common cause of nosocomial infection in hospitals and intensive care units and became more problematic as time went on. These patients were described as having risk factors of health care exposure, medical devices, older age, and other disease comorbidities. Community-associated MRSA infection has significantly different epidemiology. It was first described in 1993 in Australian aborigines without any contact with a health care system. In the United States in 1999, the Centers for Disease Control and Prevention (CDC) reported 4 rapidly fatal cases of MRSA in otherwise healthy children in the upper Midwest. Since that time, MRSA has become a well-established pathogen in the community, causing skin and soft tissue infection as well as invasive disease. Community-associated strains are generally distinguishable from health care-associated strains as they are more susceptible to most non-beta lactam antimicrobials and carry specific genes including one that encodes for a cytotoxin known as Panton-Valentine leukocidin (PVL). PVL causes most community-associated strains to cause skin and soft tissue infections. The CDC has attempted to examine the total burden of MRSA disease in the United States. In 2005, there were about 14 million outpatient health care visits for suspected SA skin infections in the United States, and extrapolating from data 1 year prior, approximately 59% were likely secondary to MRSA of the community-associated

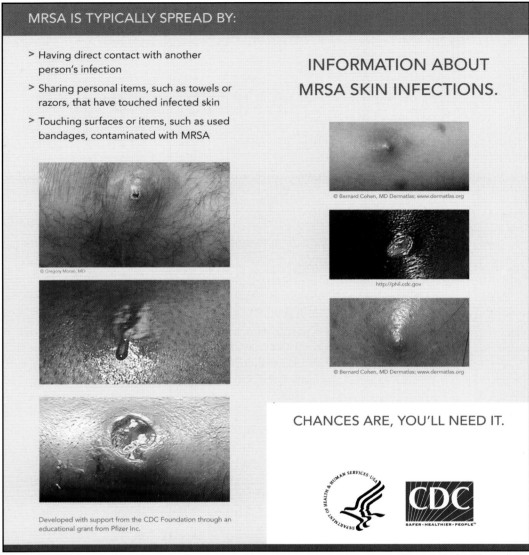

Figure 7-1. Spread of MRSA colonization and infection person to person. (Reprinted with permission of the Centers for Disease Control and Prevention. MRSA; 2010. www.cdc.gov/mrsa/library/mrsa_provider_info.html.)

variety. In that same year, about 94,000 people developed invasive disease due to MRSA and 19,000 died. Health care-associated disease may also account for some skin and soft tissue infections; however in more invasive disease, health care-associated infections are a much greater burden than community-associated infections as they account for 86% of severe infections. Health care-associated infections are subcategorized into hospital-onset and community-onset depending on where they originate.

How is MRSA spread (Figure 7-1)? As MRSA is widespread in the community, anyone is at risk for becoming colonized. Colonization does not necessarily result in infection.

Risk factors for infection include cuts or broken skin, skin-to-skin contact, contaminated surfaces, crowded living conditions, and poor hygiene. Person-to-person transmission was the predominant mode of spread in outbreaks in several populations. These include inmates, military personnel, athletes, intravenous drug users, day care attendees, dormitories, men who have sex with men, heterosexual couples, and medically underserved populations. Other epidemiologic risk factors have also been suggested in the literature including age younger than 2 years or older than 65 years, persons living in residential homes or shelters, veterinarians, pet owners, pig farmers, Blacks, recent influenza infection, history of colonization or recent infection with MRSA, and household contact with a MRSA colonized or infected person.

Outbreaks of MRSA in athletes have occurred and been highlighted in the press. CDC investigated an outbreak among the members of the St. Louis Rams football team during the 2003 season. They found 8 MRSA infections in 5 players that were significantly associated with linebacker or lineman position as well as higher body mass index. The infected players were all close to each other in their positions on the field and in the locker room. All of the infections developed at turf abrasion sites. Interestingly, an indistinguishable MRSA strain was found in a competing team as well as in other regions around the United States.

Since that time, several outbreaks in athletic teams have been described including younger athletes. These have been associated with sports that involve skin-to-skin contact and frequent skin abrasions, predominantly wrestling, football, and rugby, but cases have occurred among athletes in other sports, including soccer, basketball, field hockey, volleyball, rowing, martial arts, fencing, and baseball. The CDC provides resources for athletic teams, coaches, and players for prevention and treatment of MRSA infection.

Should schools be concerned? The daily routine of school generally does not put students at higher risk than anywhere else in the community. In contrast to the experience in contact sports, spread in classrooms has not been a recognized problem. Administrators may be pressured to take drastic measures when cases of MRSA occur in a school, such as to close schools to perform disinfection of the entire school. This is not necessary.

Prevention of transmission is best achieved by good hygiene. Hand washing with soap and water or an alcohol-based hand rub is the most important form of prevention. Other important strategies include keeping cuts and scrapes clean and covered, avoidance of other people's wounds, not sharing personal items such as towels or razors, and keeping athletic equipment clean. Persons with MRSA infections should be instructed to keep their wound covered and dry and to routinely clean off frequently touched surfaces. Routine cleaning with disinfectants that are known to kill SA on areas that are likely to have been contacted by uncovered or poorly covered infections is appropriate. If there are multiple cases, consultation with the local health department may help aid in decision making for administrators. It is not recommended that schools inform the entire student body about one case of MRSA infection in the school. More specific recommendations are available that deal with athletic facilities, athletic equipment, towels, and other surfaces that may come into contact with athletes' bare skin.

Suggested Readings

Boucher HW, Corey GR. Epidemiology of methicillin-resistant *Staphylococcus aureus*. *Clin Infect Dis*. 2008;46(suppl 5): s344-s349.

Centers for Disease Control and Prevention. MRSA Infections. http://www.cdc.gov/mrsa/index.html

Kazakova SV, Hagrman JC, Matava M, et al. A clone of methicillin-resistant *Staphylococcus aureus* among professional football players. *N Engl J Med*. 2005;352(5):468-475.

Klevens RM, Morrison MA, Nadle J, et al. Invasive methicillin-resistant *Staphylococcus aureus* infections in the United States. *JAMA*. 2007;298(15):1763-1771.

ARE THERE ENVIRONMENTAL CLEANING OR PERSONAL HYGIENE INTERVENTIONS THAT CAN BE USED TO REDUCE RECURRENCES OF METHICILLIN-RESISTANT STAPHYLOCOCCUS AUREUS INFECTIONS?

Emily A. Thorell, MD

Most recurrences methicillin-resistant *Staphylococcus aureus* (MRSA) infections arise from organisms that colonize the patient's nares, axilla, groin, or other sites. It is unknown whether environmental cleaning interventions will actually reduce recurrences of MRSA infections. Environmental contamination may play an important role in transmission within households and might allow reinfection after decolonization.

MRSA infections linked to environmental sources have been reported since before the emergence of community-associated MRSA (CA-MRSA). Contamination of fomites has been described in many settings. Stethoscopes, pagers, bed spaces, and workstations have been found to be colonized with *S aureus* (SA), including MRSA, in hospitals. SA, including MRSA, has also been cultured from household areas that are commonly touched such as toilet handles, sinks, and doorknobs, and has been implicated in contributing to recurrent infection. Athletic gear and equipment used by athletes such as benches, uniforms, bar soap, whirlpools, shared towels, and razors have been implicated in transmission as well. Ultimately, MRSA may be anywhere; therefore, environmental cleaning is a strategy that may be useful to decrease transmission in households that have people who are infected or colonized with MRSA, but it is unclear if this will decrease recurrences.

In the hospital setting, routine infection control measures such as standard precautions for all patients and contact precautions (gown and gloves with or without eye protection if needed) for those who are known/suspected to be colonized or infected with MRSA are recommended. In addition, updated guidelines were recently published by the Centers for Disease Control and Prevention (CDC) for use in the outpatient setting. These recommendations discuss the particulars of hand hygiene, personal protective equipment, and environmental cleaning in the setting of potential contact with bodily fluids as well as approved cleaning solutions. Finally, recommendations regarding the importance of training of health care workers in infection prevention and control practices are provided.

Personal hygiene is very important to prevent MRSA transmission (see Question 7); however, there are still no data for this intervention on recurrence. MRSA recurrences are frustrating for both clinicians and patients. Hygiene measures, decolonization of patients and family members (see Question 6), and environmental cleaning are often attempted but there is limited evidence on which modalities actually work. It makes sense that hygiene and environmental measures may prevent reinfection once a patient has been decolonized, but if other household members remain colonized, MRSA may continue to spread. Treatment with antimicrobials has not been shown to reduce recurrences and is generally not recommended (see Question 5), although this is often attempted. It is clear that more research needs to be done to understand the epidemiology and causes of CA-MRSA recurrences in order to develop better interventions. Ultimately, a vaccine against SA would be ideal, but this has not been achieved.

Patients may have questions regarding which product to use for cleaning when MRSA is a concern. It is important to understand the difference between detergents, sanitizers, and disinfectants. Soaps and detergents lift matter, including bacteria, from a surface and are used for routine cleaning. Sanitizers (ie, alcohol hand sanitizer) will reduce the amount of bacteria to nonharmful levels but may not totally eradicate them. Disinfectants are regulated by the Environmental Protection Agency and will actually kill or inactivate germs to prevent growth but have no effect on dirt or dust. Disinfectants are used for cleaning surfaces with blood or body fluid residue such as pus. These are the mainstay for use against MRSA, and patients can find these disinfectants in grocery stores labeled as effective against SA. Many clinicians recommend using disinfectants in the home to clean areas contaminated by wound drainage and high-touch areas in conjunction with other measures. Routine laundering procedures are adequate to make towels, clothes, and other linens safe to touch and wear. There are still no data as to whether home environmental cleaning prevents or decreases MRSA recurrences.

Patient education is critical—first to recognize a possible MRSA infection, and second to know what to do and when to seek medical care. The CDC has created a National MRSA Education Initiative to do just this. There is free information for patients and families as well as public service announcements easily found on the Web site. There is also a wealth of information for health care providers to use in these efforts. Use of this material is free and encouraged.

Many clinicians have compiled sets of recommendations to give to patients and their families. These are largely based on expert opinion, with some evidence as outlined in the previous 3 questions. Unfortunately, expert opinion is the highest level of evidence we have to base many of these decisions. An example is shown in Table 8-1.

Table 8-1

Key Messages for Patients With Skin and Soft Tissue Infections and Their Close Contacts

1. Keep wounds that are draining covered with clean, dry bandages.
2. Clean hands regularly with soap and water or alcohol-based hand gel (if hands are not visibly soiled). Always clean hands immediately after touching infected skin or any item that has come in direct contact with a draining wound.
3. Maintain good general hygiene with regular bathing. Wear loose fitting clothing and keep nails trimmed.
4. Do not share items that may become contaminated, such as towels, clothing, bedding, bar soap, razors, toothbrushes, and athletic equipment that touches the skin.
5. Launder clothing that has come in contact with wound drainage after each use and dry thoroughly.
6. If you are not able to keep your wound covered with a clean, dry bandage at all times, do not participate in activities where you have skin-to-skin contact with other persons (such as athletic activities) until your wound is healed.
7. Clean equipment and other environmental surfaces with which multiple individuals have bare skin contact with over the counter detergent/disinfectant that specifies SA on the product label and is suitable for the type of surface being cleaned.
8. Add ½ cup bleach to ¼-filled tub of bath water 2 to 3 times a week and soak for 15 minutes for at least 6 weeks. Chlorhexidine or hexachlorophene soap (Hibiclens [Norcross, GA] or Phisohex [Sanofi-Synthelabo Inc, Bridgewater, NJ]) may be used as an alternative but should also be left on the skin for at least 5 minutes.
9. Apply mupirocin ointment to both nares of all household family members twice daily for 5 days. Do not use for longer periods or resistance may develop, but this can be done repeatedly with recurrences.
10. Call or visit your physician if you have a new infection, as repeat culture may be helpful.

**It is very important to start household cleaning, bleach or Hibiclens/Phisohex baths, and Mupirocin on the same day for all household members. At the same time, discard old razors and toothbrushes and start with clean linens.

Suggested Readings

Begier EM, Frenette K, Barrett NL, et al. A high-morbidity outbreak of methicillin-resistant *Staphylococcus aureus* among players on a college football team, facilitated by cosmetic body shaving and turf burns. *Clin Infect Dis.* 2004;39(10):1446-1453.

Centers for Disease Control and Prevention. MRSA infections. http://www.cdc.gov/mrsa/index.html

Centers for Disease Control and Prevention. MRSA infections http://www.cdc.gov/HAI/prevent/prevent_pubs.html

Miller LG, Diep BA. Colonization, fomites, and virulence: rethinking the pathogenesis of community-associated methicillin-resistant *Staphylococcus aureus* infection. *Clin Infect Dis.* 2008;46:752-760.

Singh D, Kaur H, Gardner WG, Treen LB. Bacterial contamination of hospital pagers. *Infect Control Hosp Epidemiol.* 2002;23(5):274-276.

Smith MA, Mathewson JJ, Ulert IA, Scerpella EG, Ericsson CD. Contaminated stethoscopes revisited. *Arch Intern Med.* 1996;156(1):82-84.

Uhlemann AC, Knox J, Miller M, et al. The environment as an unrecognized reservoir for community-associated methicillin resistant *Staphylococcus aureus* USA300: a case control study. *PLoS One.* 2011;6(7):e22407.

SECTION III

TINEA CAPITIS

How Long Does Tinea Capitis Need to Be Treated in Order to Be Sure the Infection Has Cleared?

Jennifer Goldman, MD and Susan Abdel-Rahman, PharmD

In contrast to dermatophyte infections of the glabrous skin, groin, and feet, topical anti-fungal therapy alone is inadequate when treating tinea capitis as topical medications do not adequately penetrate the hair shaft where the fungus resides. The standard drug regimen for the treatment of tinea capitis in the pediatric population is a 6- to 8-week course of high-dose griseofulvin given once daily. Other orally available therapies that have been investigated include terbinafine, fluconazole, and itraconazole. Adjunctive therapies including topical shampoos (eg, selenium sulfide, ketoconazole) have also been used to minimize spore shedding during treatment.

Griseofulvin impairs the division and replication of fungal cells and binds to human keratin, inhibiting fungal invasion. The drug is not retained to any great extent in the skin and stratum corneum and this property, coupled with its fungistatic mechanism of action, necessitates prolonged treatment courses, making adherence difficult. Cost is also an issue as 6 to 8 weeks of therapy can be costly and tablets cannot be crushed, requiring a liquid formulation be dispensed to children who are unable to swallow solid dosage forms. Given the erratic absorption profile of griseofulvin, the drug is best delivered with a high-fat meal. It is approved for children older than 2 years. Adverse effects include gastrointestinal upset, rash, and headache but are rarely seen in children when the antifungal is taken for less than 8 weeks. Although griseofulvin is the drug of choice in the treatment of tinea capitis, clinical effectiveness appears to be lower than controlled clinical trials would suggest with greater than 50% of children potentially failing to clear their infection following a single course of therapy.[1]

Terbinafine has also been evaluated as a treatment option for children with tinea capitis. Terbinafine is a fungicidal agent that inhibits squalene epoxidase, weakening the fungal cell wall. It is approved by the Food and Drug Administraion (FDA) for use in children 4 years and older with tinea capitis. Although a liquid formulation is not available,

Table 9-1

Antifungals

Drug	Advantage	Disadvantage	Common Adverse Effects	Average Cost Per Day*
Griseofulvin	• Inexpensive • Liquid available	• Prolonged treatment	• Gastrointestinal • Headache • Rash	$4.82
Terbinafine	• Shorter treatment duration	• Efficacy may vary by fungal species • No liquid available • Drug interactions with CYP2D6 substrates	• Gastrointestinal • Itching/swelling of lips	$9.25
Itraconazole	• Shorter treatment duration • Liquid available	• Not approved by the FDA for tinea capitis • Drug interactions with CYP3A4 substrates	• Headache • Rash • Gastrointestinal	$15.44
Fluconazole	• Liquid available	• Dose not established for tinea capitis • Results limited mostly to *Trichophyton tonsurans* • Not approved by the FDA for tinea capitis	• Headache • Rash • Gastrointestinal • LFT abnormalities	$8.79

*Average cost based on 20-kg child. Average wholesale price obtained from Red Book.[4]

oral granule packets do exist and the stability of an extemporaneous formulation has been reported.

Terbinafine is generally well tolerated with gastrointestinal disturbances and cutaneous reactions being the most common adverse reactions. In comparing the efficacy of griseofulvin to terbinafine in the treatment of tinea capitis caused by *Trichophyton tonsurans*, studies suggest that a 2- to 4-week course of terbinafine is at least as effective as 6 to 8 weeks of griseofulvin.[2] This reduced treatment duration can be attributed, in part, to the drugs, fungicidal mechanism of action and persistence at high concentrations in keratin-rich tissues well after drug discontinuation. Although in vitro susceptibility data suggest that terbinafine is active against *Microsporum spp*, in vivo data suggest that a 6-week course of oral terbinafine may be inadequate in treating tinea capitis caused by *Microsporum canis* (Table 9-1).

Table 9-2
Barriers to Treating Tinea Capitits

Issue	*Barriers to Treatment*
Transmission	• Asymptomatic infection rates in the school or day care setting may be very high • Difficult to eradicate fungal organisms from fomites • Disease often recurs or more likely never clears
Diagnosis	• *Trichophyton tonsurans* cannot be visualized by using a Woods lamp • Antifungal susceptibility data are not routinely gathered
Treatment	• Prolonged courses are required • Griseofulvin should be administered with the "right" foods (ie, those high in fat) • Cost • Formulation (some drugs only available in tablet form, others have unpleasant taste)

Randomized controlled clinical trials also suggest that treatment outcomes with itraconazole and fluconazole may be similar to griseofulvin when treating tinea capitis caused by *Trichophyton spp*; however, data are limited for *Microsporum* infections. Both itraconazole and fluconazole impair fungal ergosterol synthesis leading to breakdown of the fungal cell wall. The most common adverse effects include gastrointestinal disturbances, headache, dizziness, and allergic reactions. Itraconazole is available in both capsule and suspension formulation, although neither is approved by the FDA for use in cases of tinea capitis infections. Length of therapy with itraconazole in treating tinea capitis has not been determined; however, clinical trials suggest that continuous and pulse regimens result in outcomes comparable with those observed with griseofulvin. Although fluconazole is widely used in children with candidiasis, its use for tinea capitis has not been sufficiently examined and the FDA has not approved it in the use of tinea capitis (see Table 9-1).[2]

Selenium sulfide is often used as an adjunctive therapy in combination with oral antifungal therapy, although only a handful of studies are available examining its utility. In a small, randomized, controlled study comparing patients treated with oral griseofulvin alone or in combination with either a nonmedicated shampoo, clotrimazole, or selenium shampoo, biweekly selenium shampooing appeared to shorten the duration that patients had positive scalp cultures when compared to the other therapies.[3] Steroids, in combination with antifungal agents, have also been used in children with kerion (boggy, inflamed areas of the scalp), although the benefit of topical or systemic steroids is unclear. Notably, kerion can often be confused with a bacterial infection; however, antimicrobial therapy has not proven to be effective.

As mentioned above, it is difficult to truly assess the effectiveness of antifungal therapy in tinea capitis (Table 9-2). Clinical trials with limited post-treatment follow-up may overestimate the long-term ability of these drugs to clear the pathogen from the scalp. Investigators have observed that patients may remain persistently culture positive despite the resolution of symptoms (see Table 9-2). Conversely, clinical findings may persist in patients who have cleared the pathogen. Not only are new antifungals needed for the treatment of pediatric dermatophytoses, but comprehensive evaluations of the true effectiveness of existing therapies are required.

Currently, griseofulvin for 6 to 8 weeks remains first-line therapy for treatment of tinea capitis in the pediatric population, although a shorter course of terbinafine can be considered. Adjunctive selenium sulfide shampoo applied twice weekly may also prove beneficial in the infected individual and may be required by some school systems before a child can be readmitted. Importantly, repeated courses of therapy may be required in persistently infected children. In these children, the risk of adverse drug effects increases with prolonged use (after >1 month of treatment) and lab monitoring, including complete blood count and liver transaminase tests, may be warranted.

References

1. Abdel-Rahman Wright KJ, Navarre HC. Griseofulvin only modestly diminishes persistence of *Trichophyton tonsurans* on the scalp of carriers. *J Pediatr Pharmacol Ther.* 2009;14:94-99.
2. Gonzalez U, Seaton T, Bergus G, Jacobson J, Martinez-Monzon C. Systemic antifungal therapy for tinea capitis in children. *Cochrane Database Syst Rev.* 2007:CD004685.
3. Allen HB, Honig PJ, Leyden JJ, McGinley KJ. Selenium sulfide: adjunctive therapy for tinea capitis. *Pediatrics.* 1982;69:81-83.
4. Red Book. Thomson Reuters: Vol 62;2011. Current release October 2011.

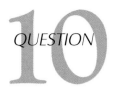

WHAT ARE THE METHODS BY WHICH TINEA CAPITIS CAN BE SPREAD FROM PERSON TO PERSON?

Jennifer Goldman, MD and Susan Abdel-Rahman, PharmD

Tinea capitis is acquired when an individual comes into direct contact with an infected person, animal, or contaminated fomite. The anthropophilic (preferring human beings) *Trichophyton tonsurans* is usually acquired from infected humans or fomites, whereas *Microsporum canis* is frequently acquired from infected cats or dogs. Importantly, infectious spores can remain viable on inanimate objects such as brushes, hats, and bedding for months to years. Dermatophyte infection rates are often higher in high-contact environments such as sports clubs, day care centers, and schools, suggesting that close contact promotes transmission of the pathogen. The spread of infection, although not completely understood, appears to differ in different settings. Genetic analyses of infecting strains from cohorts of day care center attendees, school children, and adolescents participating in club sports suggest that, in older children, infection patterns are more clonal in nature. By contrast, younger children are more likely to harbor genetic strains that are distinct from their classmates, suggesting that infection is not simply passed from person to person, but that multiple factors including a persistent carrier status play a significant role in infections of preschool-aged children.[1]

Tinea capitis, with its median infection age of 4 years, is a disease of childhood. Infection rates decrease with increasing grade level, which is likely secondary to a decrease in close contact between classmates as well as possible hormonal changes occurring during puberty that alter a child's susceptibility to infection. African Americans demonstrate the highest incidence of disease, although the reasons are not clear. It has been speculated that specific hair characteristics and/or hair care practices (eg, tight braiding) as well as lower socioeconomic status, may increase infection rates, although none of these theories have been substantiated. A large, cross-sectional surveillance study examining over 10,000 school-aged children in Kansas City confirmed that Black children had a significantly higher rate of infection (12.9%) when compared with Hispanic (1.6%) and White (1.1%) children. Although the overall infection rate in this study approximated 1 in every 15 children, more than 1 of every 8 Black children harbored *T tonsurans* and nearly 1 of every 5 in kindergarten and first grade were infected.[1]

Successful eradication of tinea capitis can be extremely difficult as this involves appropriate medical management of the infected individual in combination with environmental remediation aimed at infective fomites. In the recent past, when *Microsporum spp* were responsible for the majority of tinea capitis infections, the population at large could be easily screened with the use of an ultraviolet lamp (ie, a Woods lamp), which caused the organism to fluoresce. In the era of *T tonsurans*, screening for infected individuals is more difficult as this endothrix pathogen that invades the hair element will not fluoresce under a Woods lamp. Routine inspection of scalps would permit identification of infection in schools and day care centers, although this can be time consuming and will not identify the asymptomatic carriers, which comprise the majority of infected children.[2,3]

It is suggested that adopting good hygiene practices and minimizing the sharing of hair instruments such as combs may decrease transmission, although this is difficult to evaluate. For control measures, the American Academy of Pediatrics recommends that early treatment of infected individuals is indicated, as is the examination of household contacts for evidence of clinical infection. Children may return to school once systemic therapy has been initiated. Haircuts, shaving of the head, or wearing a cap is not necessary. The cleansing of viable spores from objects is recommended and bleach should be suitable, although higher concentrations and/or prolonged contact times may be required. Decreasing person-to-person or fomite-to-person transmission requires a multifaceted approach involving education, detection, prevention, and treatment of disease.[4]

References

1. Abdel-Rahman SM, Farrand N, Schuenemann E, et al. The prevalence of infections with *Trichophyton tonsurans* in schoolchildren: the CAPITIS study. *Pediatrics.* 2010;125(5):966-973.
2. Ilkit M, Ali Saracli M, Kurdak H, et al. Clonal outbreak of *Trichophyton tonsurans* tinea capitis gladiatorum among wrestlers in Adana, Turkey. *Med Mycol.* 2010;48(3):480-485.
3. Shinoda H, Nishimoto K, Mochizuki. Screening examination of *Trichophyton tonsurans* among judo practitioners at the all Japan inter high school championships, Saga 2007. *Nippon Ishinkin Gakkai Zasshi.* 2008;49(4):305-309.
4. Elewski BE. Tinea capitis: a current perspective. *J Am Acad Dermatol.* 2000;42(1 pt 1):1-20.

DO THERE NEED TO BE VISIBLE LESIONS TO DIAGNOSE TINEA CAPITIS?

Jennifer Goldman, MD and Susan Abdel-Rahman, PharmD

Although the clinical presentations of tinea capitis are varied, they are often recognized by the practicing clinician. Circular patches of alopecia with scaling are referred to as the "gray-type" tinea capitis. Widespread scalp scaling can also occur along with patchy hair loss, suggesting a moth-eaten appearance. A "black dot" pattern exhibits visible broken off hairs where the hair shaft has fractured secondary to dermatophyte invasion. Kerion represents an edematous, boggy localized area of inflammation. Any of these presentations may be accompanied by eczematous, papular, or pustular lesions remote from the site of infection (an Id reaction). This clinical feature represents an immune response to the fungal antigens and is devoid of organisms. Given its various forms, the differential diagnosis for tinea capitis is extensive and includes folliculitis, alopecia areata, seborrheic dermatitis, atopic dermatitis, psoriasis, and trichotillomania.

Both animals and humans can also be infected with dermatophytes yet manifest no evidence of disease. Performing scalp cultures has revealed undiagnosed cases of tinea capitis in household members of symptomatic index cases. In Philadelphia, Cleveland, and Kansas City public schools, as many as 14% of Black, school-aged children who were cultured were infected and the majority were asymptomatic. In a Kansas City preschool population, as many as 50% of cultured children were infected, significantly more than were symptomatic (Figure 11-1).[1-4]

The finding of a single positive scalp culture in the absence of symptoms should immediately prompt the question of whether the culture-positive child represents an asymptomatic carrier or whether he or she has simply transiently acquired viable fungal elements from the environment. The Philadelphia study was the first to suggest that these children might be carriers, having identified that more than half of the asymptomatic children who did not receive therapy remained culture positive 2 months after their initial evaluation.[1] The more intensive Kansas City–based preschool study went a step further and performed genetic fingerprinting on the fungal isolates that were recovered from serially culture-positive children. These investigators observed that 88% of children who were repeatedly

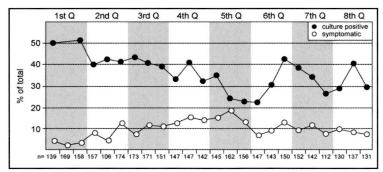

Figure 11-1. Percentage of children at each visit with a culture-positive scalp sample (closed circles) and with clinical signs and symptoms of tinea capitis (open circles). The number of children evaluated each month is provided along the x-axis. (Reproduced with permission of *Pediatrics*, Vol. 118, Pages 2365-2373, Copyright © 2006 by the AAP.)

culture positive were infected with the same genetic strain (or pair of strains) on each visit. Only 12% of the children appeared to transiently harbor the pathogen.[3]

The progression to clinically symptomatic disease is far more common in carriers as opposed to noncarriers; however, these children can remain asymptomatic for months to years, ostensibly serving as a vector of transmission to other children. As such, the recommended course of action with respect to medical management is not clear. Some investigators advocate treating all carriers with oral antimycotic agents, whereas others propose treating only those children with an arbitrarily defined "heavy" fungal load. Still others suggest that patients with "light" fungal growth may benefit from twice weekly topical shampooing using either selenium sulfide or povidone-iodine.

The practicing clinician must decide whether or not he or she would treat a carrier before screening an asymptomatic child or the close contact of an infected child. Additionally, he or she must carefully consider the risks and benefits of various treatment options before initiating therapy including issues related to cost and adherence. The assignment of risk-benefit may differ in the singular patient visiting with new-onset tinea capitis versus the patient suffering from persistent or recalcitrant infection. Although limited, there have been correlative links between asthma, atopy, and dermatophyte infections and further investigation is warranted to examine whether the treatment of fungal carriers could positively impact allergic and atopic comorbidities including asthma. Regardless of the decision to treat, education on avoiding the sharing of brushes, bedding, hats, and the like may aid in the decrease of transmission.

References

1. Williams JV, Honig PJ, McGinley KJ, Leyden JJ. Semiquantitative study of tinea capitis and the asymptomatic carrier state in inner-city school children. *Pediatrics.* 1995;96(2 pt 1):265-267.
2. Pomeranz AJ, Sabnis SS, McGrath GJ, Esterly NB. Asymptomatic dermatophyte carriers in the households of children with tinea capitis. *Arch Pediatr Adolesc Med.* 1999;153(5):483-486.
3. Abdel-Rahman SM, Simon S, Wright KJ, Ndjountche L, Gaedigk A. Tracking *Trichophyton tonsurans* through a large urban child care center: defining infection prevalence and transmission patterns by molecular strain typing. *Pediatrics.* 2006;118(6):2365-2373.
4. Ghannoum M, Isham N, Hajjeh R, et al. Tinea capitis in Cleveland: survey of elementary school students. *J Am Acad Dermatol.* 2003;48(2):189-193.

WHAT ORGANISMS ARE RESPONSIBLE FOR CAUSING TINEA CAPITIS?

Jennifer Goldman, MD and Susan Abdel-Rahman, PharmD

Cutaneous dermatophyte infections are prevalent worldwide, although infection rates and predominant fungal species vary by demographic region. *Trichophyton tonsurans* and *Microsporum canis* are currently the predominant dermatophytes in North America and much of Europe, whereas *T mentagrophytes, T rubrum, T verrucosum, T schoenleinii, T violaceum, T soudanense, T yaoundei,* and *M audouinii* are known to cause disease in other regions around the globe. For example, *T violaceum* is prevalent in Asia and Northeast Africa, whereas *T soudanense* is found in West Africa.[1] This variability of dermatophyte species based on geographical area is important to consider when treating a patient from another region of the world. Although it may not directly impact choice of therapy, it is important to recognize that various organisms may only be identified by culture depending upon a patient's travel history.[2]

During the first half of the 20th century, tinea capitis was epidemic in the United States, predominantly due to infections by species of *Microsporum*. Public health efforts were initiated to control these infections and with the introduction of griseofulvin in the late 1950s, *Microsporum*-associated infections began to wane. Since that time, *T tonsurans* has emerged as the predominate cause of tinea capitis in the United States, likely introduced by individuals migrating up through Central America and Mexico.[3] Over 65 genetically distinct strains of *T tonsurans* have been described to date and the organism now accounts for over 95% of all tinea capitis cases in the United States. Although initially restricted to North America, this particular dermatophyte species has become a major cause of infection in Western Europe, the Middle East, and Japan. Now endemic in the United States, it is unclear whether other dermatophyte species will emerge as significant contributors to tinea capitis infections.

References

1. Weitzman I, Summerbell RC. The dermatophytes. *Clin Microbiol Rev.* 1995;8(2):240-259.
2. Abdel-Rahman SM, Sugita T, Gonzalez GM, et al. Divergence among an international population of *Trichophyton tonsurans* isolates. *Mycopathologia.* 2010;169(1):1-13.
3. Frieden IJ, Howard R. Tinea capitis: epidemiology, diagnosis, treatment, and control. *J Am Acad Dermatol.* 1994;31(3 pt 2):S42-S46.

SECTION IV

TICK-BORNE ILLNESS

WHAT ARE THE BEST PROPHYLACTIC MEASURES TO TELL FAMILIES TO USE TO PREVENT TICK BITES? AT WHAT AGE ARE AGENTS SUCH AS DEET AND PICARIDIN SAFE TO USE?

Kimberly C. Martin, DO and José R. Romero, MD, FAAP

The best measures for families to use in order to prevent tick bites are reduction of environmental exposures, use of appropriate clothing, implementation of skin examination procedures, and use of repellants such as DEET (*N,N*-diethyl-meta-toluamide) and Picaridin 2-(2-hydroxyethyl)-1-piperidinecarboxylic acid 1-methylpropyl ester).

The time spent in tick-infested habitats such as tall grass, shrubs, and brush should be minimized or avoided, if possible. Children involved in hiking activities should be reminded to stay on paths and not stray into unkempt areas of the trail. Children should be dressed in light-colored clothing with long-sleeve shirts, long pants, shoes, and socks when tick bites are possible. All clothing should be tucked in, including the pants into the socks, to cover all areas where ticks could find access to the skin.

Following all outdoor activities, children should undergo a full-body skin examination to look for the presence of ticks. Special emphasis should be placed on examining the scalp, behind the ears, the axillae, the umbilicus, behind the knees, and interdigital areas of the feet. If a tick is found, it should be firmly grasped using tweezers and pulled out without squeezing. Children should be bathed within 2 hours of outdoor activities to possibly wash off any nonattached ticks missed on examination. The child's outerwear and any equipment used (ie, backpack, walking stick) should be checked for ticks to prevent transmission after arriving home. Pets that have access to the outdoors are also a potential source of tick transmission to family members. Tick repellants should be used as appropriate and pets should be checked daily for hidden ticks.

Chemoprophylactic measures for the prevention of tick bites rely on the use of repellant products such as DEET and Picaridin. Both have been studied extensively and have approval from the Environmental Protection Agency (EPA) for use in humans in order to repel insects including ticks. The American Academy of Pediatrics (AAP) has provided a greater body of recommendations for the use of DEET than for Picaridin.

Both have a range of protection of 3 to 8 hours. DEET should not be applied more than once a day in typical settings, and reapplication of Picardin is dependent upon the concentration of the repellant. Sunscreens containing DEET are not recommended for use in children. These agents are designed for direct application to the skin but should not be used around the eyes, mouth, or on open skin lesions. They should not be applied under clothing. Children should have the product applied by an adult and should not have easy access to the agents. For application on the face, the product should be sprayed into the hand of an adult and applied to the child's face. After returning home from activities in which the above agents are used, the skin should be washed with soap and water and clothing should be laundered in the normal manner.

The AAP recommends specific age minimums for the use of these agents. The use of DEET in children should be reserved for those older than or equal to 2 months. Although the formulations for use in humans range from 4% to 100% concentrations of DEET, the AAP advises the use of products containing 10% to 30% concentrations for children. Although the AAP has not issued a formal recommendation for Picaridin use in children, some AAP publications have advised that its use be reserved for children older than 6 months and that products contain 5% to 10% concentrations.

When using DEET- or Picaridin-containing products, it is necessary to follow all package directions. Although historically there were concerns about using DEET in children, these concerns were unfounded. DEET has an excellent safety profile with few side effects, when used properly. DEET does irritate mucous membranes and has caused encephalopathy in the setting of accidental ingestion. However, the most common adverse reaction is urticaria and contact dermatitis. There have been no reports of serious adverse events with Picardin. If a rash or other allergic symptoms develop after use of DEET or Picaridin, the AAP recommends that the product be washed off with soap and water and that the local poison control be contacted for further recommendations.

In addition to the above, the CDC recommends measures to create tick-free zones around homes, schools, and other play areas. Advise parents to keep their lawn clear of dead leaves and brush and to place wood chips or gravel between yards and wooded areas. Playground equipment, picnic tables, and patios should be kept away from trees and lawn edges to prevent tick infections. The CDC also advises an application of pesticides to geographically susceptible lawns at the end of May or beginning of June to reduce *Ixodes* tick populations by 68% to 100% (Figure 13-1).

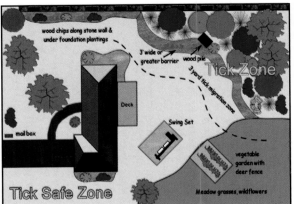

Figure 13-1. Creating a tick safe zone around a home. (Centers for Disease Control and Prevention. www.cdc.gov/ncidod/dvbid/lyme/resources/tick_info-card.pdf. Reprinted with permission of Kirby C. Stafford III, PhD.)

Suggested Readings

Centers for Disease Control and Prevention. Protect yourself from tick-borne diseases. *Lyme Disease Resources*. March 2007. Available at http://www.cdc.gov/ncidod/dvbid/lyme/resources/tick_infocard.pdf. Accessed October 26, 2010.

Roberts J, Weil W, Shannon M. DEET Alternatives considered to be effective mosquito repellents. *AAP News*. 2005; 26(6):15.

Shelov S. Insect bites and stings. Healthychildren.org [Online]. August 2010. Available at http://www.healthychildren.org/English/health-issues/conditions/skin/Pages/Insect-Bites-and-Stings.aspx. Accessed September 9, 2010.

United States Environmental Protection Agency. New Pesticide Fact Sheet-Picaridin. *Prevention, Pesticides and Toxic Substances*. May 2005. Available at http://www.epa.gov/opprd001/factsheets/picaridin.pdf. Accessed September 15, 2010.

United States Environmental Protection Agency. The Insect Repellant DEET. *Pesticides: Topical & Chemical Fact Sheets*. March 2007. Available at http://www.epa.gov/pesticides/factsheets/chemicals/deet.htm. Accessed September 15, 2010.

WHEN ARE TICK-BORNE INFECTIONS TYPICALLY SEEN IN THE UNITED STATES, AND WHEN DOES THE PEAK TIME OCCUR?

Kimberly C. Martin, DO and José R. Romero, MD, FAAP

Tick-borne infections encompass a group of tick-vectored diseases that physicians must be mindful of when evaluating a febrile child with an appropriate exposure history. The major tick-borne illnesses in North America include Lyme disease, Rocky Mountain spotted fever (RMSF), human monocytic ehrlichiosis, human granulocytic anaplasmosis, tularemia, and babesiosis. Less commonly encountered tick-borne diseases include Colorado tick fever, Powassan encephalitis, Q fever, tick-borne relapsing fever, and Southern tick-associated rash illness. Each of these diseases has a known or putative etiologic agent, tick vector(s), and geographic distribution (Figure 14-1).

Tick-borne illnesses exhibit peak prevalence in the late spring through fall, which parallels the activity of their arthropod vectors. However, cases have occurred in every month of the year and should, therefore, be included in the differential diagnosis for appropriate patients. Often the presenting signs and symptoms are vague, nonspecific (fever, malaise, myalgia, headache, and rash), and overlap with many other illnesses, making their diagnosis difficult. However, there are some clinical clues that separate these various infections, which will be mentioned with the different infecting agents.

Lyme disease is the most commonly reported tick-borne infection in the United States. The etiologic agent is *Borrelia burgdorferi*, and the infection is characterized in 3 stages. The first, or early localized, stage is recognized by an erythema migrans rash that starts as a macular or papular lesion that enlarges and develops into a large (>5 cm) area often with central clearing. The rash is often accompanied by fever, headache, malaise, neck stiffness, and myalgias and arthralgias. The second, or early disseminated stage, is represented by multiple erythema migrans lesions, meningitis, carditis, and cranial nerve VII palsy in addition to the above-mentioned features. Finally, the third or late disease stage is typically characterized by relapsing arthritis of the large joints, with rare cases of peripheral neuropathy and demyelinating encephalitis noted.

Figure 14-1. Relative sizes of various ticks at different life stages. (Reprinted with permission of the Centers for Disease Control and Prevention. www.cdc.gov/ticks/life_cycle_and_hosts.html.)

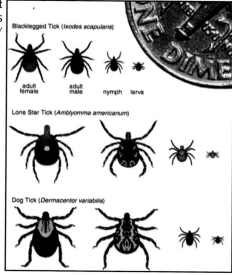

Figure 14-2. Distribution of reported cases of Lyme disease in the United States. (Reprinted with permission of the Centers for Disease Control and Prevention. www.cdc.gov/lyme/stats/maps/map2010.html)

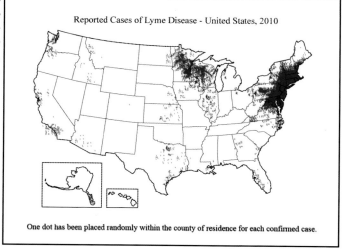

The ticks responsible for transmission are the Blacklegged tick (*Ixodes scapularis*) and the Western Blacklegged tick (*Ixodes pacificus*). Peak transmission occurs during the summer months of June, July, and August. The majority of Lyme disease cases are reported from 10 states in the Northeast and north-central portions of the United States (Connecticut, Delaware, Maryland, Massachusetts, Minnesota, New Jersey, New York, Pennsylvania, Rhode Island, and Wisconsin) (Figure 14-2). The disease is also seen on a much smaller scale on the West coast and in Alaska but is not seen in the mid-Western states in patients who have not traveled to a Lyme disease-endemic area.

RMSF was initially recognized in Montana and Idaho (Northern Rocky Mountains), but cases have occurred in almost every state in the continental United States. The causative agent is *Rickettsia rickettsii*, a gram-negative obligate intracellular coccobacillus. RMSF is a small-vessel vasculitis, which manifests with an erythematous macular rash that starts

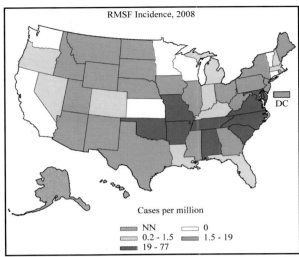

Figure 14-3. Annual incidence per million population for Rocky Mountain spotted fever, by state, in the United States for 2008. (Reprinted with permission of the Centers for Disease Control and Prevention. www.cdc.gov/rmsf/stats/)

on the wrists and ankles and generally spreads centrally with concurrent evolution into a maculopapular and petechial appearance. The palms and soles are usually involved. However, rash may not develop in up to 20% of patients. Additional features include fever, headache, myalgias, abdominal pain, vomiting, and diarrhea. Laboratory abnormalities may also be seen including hyponatremia, thrombocytopenia, and less commonly leucopenia and anemia.

The ticks known to be primary vectors of RMSF are the Rocky Mountain wood and American dog ticks (*Dermacentor andersoni* and *Dermacentor variabilis*, respectively) as well as the brown dog tick (*Rhipicephalus sanguineus*) in Arizona. Although RMSF has been reported throughout most states in the contiguous US, 60% of cases reported to the Centers for Disease Control and Prevention (CDC) were from Arkansas, Missouri, North Carolina, Oklahoma, and Tennessee (Figure 14-3). The peak incidence of disease is from April through October, but cases have been reported in every month of the year.

Human monocytic ehrlichiosis was first reported in the United States in 1986. In 1991, *Ehrlichia chaffeensis*, an obligate intracellular gram-negative organism, was documented to be a causal agent. The principal tick responsible for transmission of *Ehrlichia chaffeensis* is the Lone star tick (*Amblyomma americanum*), although the American dog and Western Blacklegged ticks are also capable of transmitting it. Cases are reported primarily from 7 states, including Arkansas, Georgia, Maryland, Missouri, North Carolina, Oklahoma, and Tennessee (Figure 14-4). The peak period of disease correlates with the highest tick activity in April through September.

Anaplasmosis, which was once referred to as human granulocytic ehrlichiosis, is now noted to be a distinct entity and is also known as human granulocytic anaplasmosis. The majority of clinical manifestations of this infection are identical to ehrlichiosis, and generally manifest as fever, myalgias, headache, and nausea. A variable appearing rash that spares the hands and feet manifests in 60% of children with ehrlichiosis and only 10% of children with anaplasmosis. Laboratory abnormalities are commonly seen and include leukopenia, thrombocytopenia, and transaminitis.

Figure 14-4. Incidence of ehrlichiosis (caused by *E chaffeensis*) by state, as reported to the CDC in 2008. (Reprinted with permission of the Centers for Disease Control and Prevention. www.cdc.gov/Ehrlichiosis/stats/)

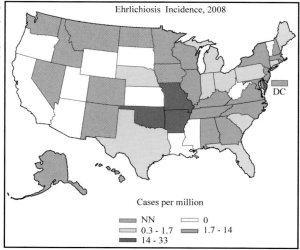

Figure 14-5. Reported cases of tularemia-United States, 2001-2010. (Reprinted with permission of the Centers for Disease Control and Prevention. www.cdc.gov/tularemia/statistics/map.html)

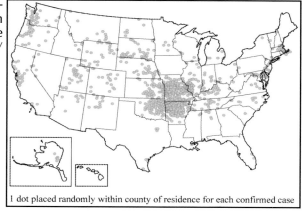

Tularemia is seen primarily in the southern states of Arkansas, Missouri, and Oklahoma but has been reported in all states except Hawaii (Figure 14-5). Although the causative agent, *Francisella tularensis*, may be transmitted through routes other than a tick bite, of the cases from Missouri reported to the CDC in 2000–2007 for which an exposure source was documented, approximately 70% were tick related. The most common form of tularemia is the ulceroglandular form, as evidenced by an ulcer developing at the site of the tick bite and an enlarged lymph node(s) at a nearby site draining the corresponding region. The second most common form is the glandular form without an associated ulcer, and less commonly oculoglandular, oropharyngeal, pneumonic, and typhoidal forms occur. The specific tick vectors include the Lone star tick and the Dog tick. The peak period of illness also follows a vernal distribution of May through September.

Babesiosis is also transmitted primarily during the summer months of May through September by the same tick that transmits Lyme disease—The Blacklegged tick. Human babesiosis is caused by the intraerythrocytic parasite *Babesia microti*. This illness is primarily seen in the New England region, and although not well studied in children, appears to have similar rates of infection in children and adults. Characteristics of babesiosis include a prodromal illness with malaise and anorexia, followed by development of fever with hemolytic anemia. However, clinical signs are generally minimal, making a detailed history and high index of suspicion key in determining this diagnosis. Untreated patients may continue to have a persistent low-level parasitemia for more than 1 year.

Suggested Readings

American Academy of Pediatrics. Babesiosis. In: Pickering LK, Baker CJ, Kimberlin DW, Long SS, eds. *Red Book: 2009 Report of the Committee on Infectious Diseases.* 28th ed. Elk Grove Village, IL: American Academy of Pediatrics; 2009:226-227.

American Academy of Pediatrics. Ehrlichia and anaplasma infections. In: Pickering LK, Baker CJ, Kimberlin DW, Long SS, eds. *Red Book: 2009 Report of the Committee on Infectious Diseases.* 28th ed. Elk Grove Village, IL: American Academy of Pediatrics; 2009:284-287.

American Academy of Pediatrics. Lyme disease. In: Pickering LK, Baker CJ, Kimberlin DW, Long SS, eds. *Red Book: 2009 Report of the Committee on Infectious Diseases.* 28th ed. Elk Grove Village, IL: American Academy of Pediatrics; 2009:430-435.

American Academy of Pediatrics. Rocky Mountain spotted fever. In: Pickering LK, Baker CJ, Kimberlin DW, Long SS, eds. *Red Book: 2009 Report of the Committee on Infectious Diseases.* 28th ed. Elk Grove Village, IL: American Academy of Pediatrics; 2009:573-575.

American Academy of Pediatrics. Tularemia. In: Pickering LK, Baker CJ, Kimberlin DW, Long SS, eds. *Red Book: 2009 Report of the Committee on Infectious Diseases.* 28th ed. Elk Grove Village, IL: American Academy of Pediatrics; 2009:708-710.

Krause PJ, Telford SR, Pollack RJ, et al. Babesiosis: an underdiagnosed disease of children. *Pediatrics.* 1992;89(6): 1045-1048.

Murphree Bacon R, Kugeler K, Mead P. Surveillance for Lyme Disease—United States, 1992-2006. *MMWR Surveill Summ.* 2008;57(SS10):1-9.

Razzaq S, Schutze GE. Rocky Mountain spotted fever: a physician's challenge. *Pediatr Rev.* 2005;26(4):125-130.

Schutze GE. Ehrlichiosis. *Pediatr Infect Dis J.* 2006;25(1):71-72.

Tularemia-Missouri, 2000-2007. *MMWR Weekly.* 2009;58(11):744-748.

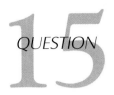

WHAT IS THE BEST EMPIRIC AND/OR PROPHYLACTIC THERAPY FOR A CHILD IN WHOM YOU SUSPECT A TICK-BORNE INFECTION?

Kimberly C. Martin, DO and José R. Romero, MD, FAAP

When selecting the most appropriate antimicrobial agent for empiric therapy of a child in whom a tick-borne infection is suspected, it is necessary to consider factors such as the geographic distribution of the specific organisms, the time of year, travel history, and the nature of the exposure. Consideration of these factors may help identify the most likely tick-borne agent(s) that could be the cause of the child's clinical syndrome under evaluation. However, even when using this approach, it is often not possible to narrow the potential cause to a single agent. It is, therefore, reassuring to know that for 4 of the most common tick-borne infections encountered in North America (Lyme disease, Rocky Mountain spotted fever [RMSF], human monocytic ehrlichiosis [HME], and tularemia), reasonable empiric coverage can be provided using a single antibiotic—doxycycline—while establishing a definitive diagnosis. This holds true even for children younger than 8 years when RMSF is suspected or is a reasonable possibility based on exposure history.

Signs and symptoms of RMSF begin after an incubation period of approximately 7 days (range from 2 days to 2 weeks). Clinical symptoms are initially vague and may mimic those of a "viral infection" with complaints of fever, nausea, vomiting, headache, decreased appetite, and general malaise. After 2 to 4 days, a blanching macular erythematous rash may appear in the majority of pediatric cases (Figure 15-1). The rash initially involves the ankles, feet, wrists, and hands, notably without sparing of the palms and soles. The rash quickly spreads to the trunk and head. The rash becomes petechial in approximately 50% of cases. Abdominal pain may be present and severe enough to mimic that of acute appendicitis or other abdominal surgical emergencies. Neurologic symptoms may include severe headache, altered mental status, or meningismus and, on occasion, seizures, cranial nerve palsies, and coma. Critically ill patients may show signs of disseminated intravascular coagulation or other acute pulmonary involvement such as pulmonary edema or acute respiratory distress syndrome.

Figure 15-1. Rocky Mountain spotted fever rash. (Reprinted with permission of the Centers for Disease Control and Prevention. Diagnosis and management of tick-borne rickettsial diseases: Rocky Mountain spotted fever, ehrlichioses, and anaplasmosis—United States: a practical guide for physicians and other health care and public health professionals. www.cdc.gov/rmsf/symptoms/index.html.)

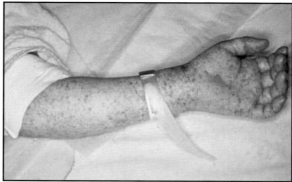

Figure 15-2. Ulceroglandular tularemia lesion. (Reprinted with permission of José R. Romero, MD.)

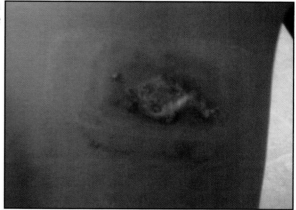

Because of the potential for significant mortality and morbidity associated with delayed initiation of the therapy for RMSF, therapy should *never* be withheld while awaiting results of confirmatory testing for this condition. Empiric therapy for all children, *regardless of age*, for suspected RMSF should begin immediately with orally or intravenously administered doxycycline (2 mg/kg/dose twice daily, maximum 100 mg/dose). Treatment should be continued until the child remains fever free for 3 days.

The signs and symptoms of HME may be similar to those seen with RMSF and include fever, headache, myalgia, decreased appetite, and abdominal pain. A macular, maculopapular, or petechial rash most prominent on the trunk is observed in two-thirds of cases. Laboratory findings are significant for hyponatremia, thrombocytopenia, elevated liver function tests, and leukopenia. Treatment of HME is similar to that of RMSF: doxycycline (2 mg/kg/dose twice daily, maximum 100 mg/dose). The duration of treatment should continue for 3 days after sustained defervescence.

The most common clinical syndrome associated with tick-borne tularemia is the ulceroglandular syndrome. The onset of the illness follows an average incubation period of 3 to 4 days (range 1 to 21 days). It is characterized by the abrupt onset of high fever, headache, chills, myalgia, anorexia, and emesis. Approximately 2 days after the onset of the nonspecific constitutional signs and symptoms, the child may complain of tender regional lymphadenopathy. Shortly thereafter, a papular lesion develops distal to the

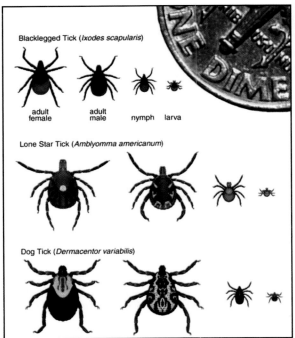

Figure 15-3. Relative sizes of various ticks at different life stages. (Reprinted with permission of the Centers for Disease Control and Prevention. www.cdc.gov/ticks/life_cycle_and_hosts.html.)

involved regional lymph nodes and progresses ultimately to ulceration (Figure 15-2). The involved lymph nodes may drain spontaneously. The fever, ulcer, and lymphadenopathy may persist for several weeks.

For children, the traditionally recommended antibiotic for therapy is streptomycin, 15 mg/kg IM twice daily (maximum dosage 2 g/d) for 7 days. However, recently, this antibiotic has become difficult to obtain. Alternative antibiotic choices include gentamicin, 2.5 mg/kg IM or IV twice daily, or doxycycline. The latter may be used in children younger than 8 years if the pharmacologic benefit outweighs the potential adverse effect of teeth staining. For children greater than 45 kg, doxycycline 100 mg IV twice daily or if less than 45 kg, doxycycline 2 mg/kg IV twice daily is recommended. In deciding whether to use gentamicin or doxycycline, it is important to recognize that relapse rates are higher following the use of doxycycline. Patients receiving streptomycin or gentamicin should be monitored for hearing loss.

The clinical manifestations of the various stages of Lyme disease are described elsewhere (see Question 16) as well as the recommendations for therapy. However, patients and families often ask about prophylactic therapy to prevent infection in the setting of a known tick bite in a Lyme endemic area. Practice guidelines published by the Infectious Diseases Society of America (IDSA) have strongly recommended against antimicrobial prophylaxis following a recognized tick bite. Nevertheless, if prophylaxis is desired, doxycycline is the sole recommended drug for this purpose. Furthermore, all 4 criteria must be met:

- The tick can be reliably identified as an adult or nymphal *Ixodes scapularis* tick. The tick must have been attached for an estimated period of more than or equal to 36 hours based on the degree of engorgement or on the time of exposure to the tick. This requires that health care providers have training in identifying *I scapularis* ticks and their multiple stages (Figure 15-3) and recognizing partially engorged ticks.

- Prophylaxis can be started within 72 hours from time of removal of the tick.
- The local rate of infection of *I scapularis* with *Borrelia burgdorferi* is more than or equal to 20%.
- Use of doxycycline is not contraindicated.

If all of the above criteria are met, a single dose of doxycycline 4 mg/kg, maximum dose 200 mg, can be given to children older than 8 years. The use of doxycycline is relatively contraindicated in children younger than 8 years. The IDSA guidelines state that no acceptable antibiotic substitution has been studied for children younger than 8 years.

Babesia microti may result in asymptomatic infection in approximately 50% of children. The disease can be rapidly fatal in immunocompromised patients. The incubation period ranges from 1 to several weeks. The onset of symptoms is gradual and includes fatigue and malaise. Fever may be high and associated with chills, myalgia, nausea, vomiting, and anorexia. In severe cases, patients may experience respiratory failure, disseminated intravascular coagulation (DIC), cardiac failure, and renal failure.

Babesiosis is treated using various combinations of antimicrobials. For less severe disease, atovaquone plus azithromycin or clindamycin may be administered for 7 to 10 days. In those with severe illness, quinine and intravenously administered clindamycin is recommended. Additionally, exchange transfusion should be considered as an adjunctive measure. Dosages include atovaquone 40 mg/kg/day orally divided every 12 hours (maximum dose 750 mg/dose), azithromycin 12 mg/kg/day orally once daily (maximum dose 600 mg/dose), clindamycin 20 to 40 mg/kg/day intravenously or orally divided every 8 hours (maximum dose 900 mg/dose), and quinine 30 mg/kg/day orally divided every 8 hours (maximum dose 650 mg/dose).

Suggested Readings

American Academy of Pediatrics. Babesiosis. In: Pickering LK, Baker CJ, Kimberlin DW, Long SS, eds. *Red Book: 2009 Report of the Committee on Infectious Diseases*. 28th ed. Elk Grove Village, IL: American Academy of Pediatrics; 2009:226-227.

American Academy of Pediatrics. Tularemia. In: Pickering LK, Baker CJ, Kimberlin DW, Long SS, eds. *Red Book: 2009 Report of the Committee on Infectious Diseases*. 28th ed. Elk Grove Village, IL: American Academy of Pediatrics; 2009:708-710.

Razzaq S, Schutze GE. Rocky Mountain spotted fever: a physician's challenge. *Pediatr Rev*. 2005;26(4):125-130.

Schutze GE. Ehrlichiosis. *Pediatr Infect Dis J*. 2006;25(5):71-72.

Tularemia-Missouri, 2000-2007. *MMWR Weekly*. 2009;58(27):744-748.

Wormser R, Dattwyler R, Shapiro E, et al. The clinical assessment, treatment, and prevention of Lyme disease, human granulocytic anaplasmosis, and babesiosis: clinical practice guidelines by the Infectious Diseases Society of America. *Clin Infect Dis*. 2006;43(9):1089-1134.

IN WHAT PARTS OF THE UNITED STATES IS LYME DISEASE SEEN, HOW IS DIAGNOSIS CONFIRMED, AND WHAT IS THE APPROPRIATE TREATMENT?

Kimberly C. Martin, DO and José R. Romero, MD, FAAP

Lyme disease is the most commonly reported tick-borne illness in the United States. Infections predominantly occur in the Northeast and north-central portions of the United States (Figure 16-1). Ninety-three percent of infections reported to the Centers for Disease Control and Prevention (CDC) from 1992 to 2006 were reported in 10 states: Connecticut, Delaware, Maryland, Massachusetts, Minnesota, New Jersey, New York, Pennsylvania, Rhode Island, and Wisconsin. The Pacific Northwest states also have a moderate number of Lyme disease cases, but this region in not considered by the CDC to be endemic for the disease. In addition to the United States, Lyme disease has also been reported in Europe and Asia. The geographic restriction of the disease is the result of the ecologic niche required for the vectors, the Blacklegged tick (*Ixodes scapularis*) and the Western Blacklegged tick (*Ixodes pacificus*).

The disease was first recognized in 1975 after a cluster of arthritis cases occurred in children living near Lyme, Connecticut. *Borrelia burgdorferi* was subsequently determined to be the etiologic agent of Lyme disease. Ticks that become infected with *B burgdorferi* acquire the spirochete through feeding on sylvatic animals such as white-footed mice and white-tailed deer, which are the principal reservoirs for the *Borrelia spp.* Epizootic transmission occurs when ticks subsequently transmit the infection to humans while feeding.

Lyme disease can be divided into 3 temporally based stages. The common manifestations of early (first stage) Lyme disease include a characteristic rash called erythema migrans, which is identified as a spreading erythematous rash with or without central clearing (Figure 16-2). On average, the skin lesion lasts approximately 3 weeks. The rash is often accompanied by fever, headache, myalgia, fatigue, arthralgia, and stiff neck. Left untreated the disease may progress to more serious neurologic (meningitis, meningoencephalitis, uni- or bilateral facial palsy, etc) or cardiac (atrioventricular heart

Figure 16-1. Distribution of reported cases of Lyme disease in the United States. (Reprinted with permission of the Centers for Disease Control and Prevention. www.cdc.gov/lyme/stats/maps/map2010.html.)

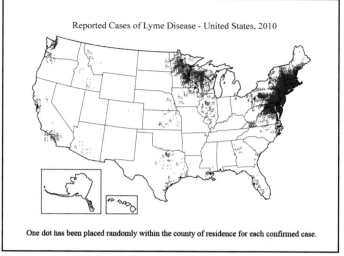

Reported Cases of Lyme Disease - United States, 2010

One dot has been placed randomly within the county of residence for each confirmed case.

Figure 16-2. Erythema migrans rash. (Reprinted with permission of the Centers for Disease Control and Prevention. www.cdc.gov/ticks/symptoms.htm. Image taken by James Gathany.)

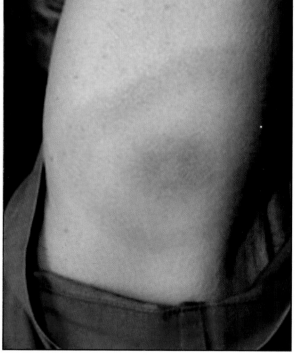

block, myocarditis) manifestations termed early disseminated (second stage). The infection may ultimately result in arthritis in half of infected individuals if not treated. The arthritis tends to involve large joints (knee, shoulder, elbow, etc) with a sudden onset. The involved joint is tender, swollen, and warm.

The diagnosis of Lyme disease may be made clinically and confirmed serologically. If the patient presents with erythema migrans and a history of tick exposure, the diagnosis can be based solely on the clinical presentation. However, if the patient presents later in the course of illness, serologic testing is necessary.

The CDC recommends a two-phased diagnostic approach consisting of an initial enzyme-linked immunosorbent assay (ELISA) followed by a specific Western blot assay. If the initial ELISA is negative, further validation is unnecessary. If the ELISA result is positive or indeterminate, additional confirmatory testing using Western blot is indicated. A Western blot assay detecting both IgM and IgG should be performed if the child is being evaluated within 4 weeks of symptom onset. Children with clinically suspected early (Stage 1) disease who test negative should undergo paired acute and convalescent serologic testing. The IgG Western blot may be performed without the IgM component after 4 weeks of symptoms because most patients with disseminated (later stages) disease will have IgG present.

Interpretation of the Western blot assay is based on the number of bands detected for each of the immunoglobulin isotypes. The IgM Western blot result is considered positive if 2 of the 3 bands tested are present. In the case of the IgG Western blot, the result is designated as positive if 5 of the 10 bands tested for are present.

Currently recommended oral antibiotics for the treatment of erythema migrans (early disease) or early disseminated disease in children include use of one of the orally administered antibiotics listed in Table 16-1.

Because macrolides have not been proven to be as effective in treating Lyme disease, they should only be used when children are intolerant or allergic to the primary medications. Close clinical observation should be provided to ensure resolution of the symptoms of Lyme disease. Repeat serologic testing is not indicated.

Other more serious manifestations of Lyme disease include meningitis, cardiac disease (early disseminated disease), and arthritis (late Lyme disease). These more severe manifestations of Lyme disease should be treated with oral or, in certain cases, parenteral therapy (Table 16-2). For detailed discussions concerning therapeutic options for these and other conditions, consult the IDSA Practice Guidelines (see reference).

Table 16-1
Therapy for Early Localized Lyme Disease

Antibiotic	Dose (mg/kg/d)	Dosing Interval	Maximum Dose Per Interval	Duration of Therapy (Days)	Indication
Amoxicillin§	50	3 divided doses	500 mg	14 to 21	<8 years
Doxycycline§	4	2 divided doses	100 mg	14 to 21	>8 years
Cefuroxime axetil§*	30	2 divided doses	500 mg	14 to 21	<8 years
Azithromycinʃ	10	Once daily	500 mg	14 to 21	*Penicillin or cephalosporin allergy or intolerance*
Clarithromycinʃ	7.5	Twice daily	500 mg	14 to 21	*Penicillin or cephalosporin allergy or intolerance*
Erythromycinʃ	12.5	Every 6 hours	500 mg	14 to 21	*Penicillin or cephalosporin allergy or intolerance*

Information derived from §AAP Red Book[1] and ʃIDSA Clinical Practice Guidelines[2]
*Alternative for amoxicillin.
Bolded italicized text denotes second-line therapy

References

1. American Academy of Pediatrics. Lyme disease. In: Pickering LK, Baker CJ, Kimberlin DW, Long SS, eds. *Red Book: 2009 Report of the Committee on Infectious Diseases.* 28th ed. Elk Grove Village, IL: American Academy of Pediatrics; 2009:430-435.
2. Wormser R, Dattwyler R, Shapiro E, et al. The clinical assessment, treatment, and prevention of Lyme disease, human granulocytic anaplasmosis, and babesiosis: Clinical Practice Guidelines by the Infectious Diseases Society of America. *Clin Infect Dis.* 2006;43(9):1089-1134.

Suggested Readings

Murphree Bacon R, Kugeler K, Mead P. Surveillance for Lyme disease—United States, 1992-2006. *MMWR Surveill Summ.* 2008;57(SS10):1-9.
Notice to Readers Recommendations for Test Performance and Interpretation from the Second National Conference on Serologic Diagnosis of Lyme Disease. *MMWR Weekly.* 1995;44(31):590-591.

Table 16-2

Antibiotic Treatment Regimens for Early Disseminated and Late Lyme Disease

Disease Manifestation	Medication	Dosage	Dosing Interval	Maximum Dose	Duration of Therapy (Days)	Route of Administration
Meningitis						
	Ceftriaxone	75 to 100 mg/kg/day	Once daily	2 g/day	14 to 28	IV
	Penicillin G	300,000 units/kg/day	6 divided doses	20 million units/day	14 to 28	IV
Lyme facial nerve palsy						
	Same regimen as early localized Lyme disease (see Table 16-1) for 21 to 28 days.					
Lyme arthritis						
	Amoxicillin	50 mg/kg/day	3 divided doses	500 mg/dose	28	PO
	Cefuroxime axetil	30 mg/kg/day	2 divided doses	500 mg/dose	28	PO
	Doxycycline	4 mg/kg/day	2 divided doses	200 mg/day	28	PO
Lyme carditis						
	Ceftriaxone	75 to 100 mg/kg/day	Once daily	2 g/day	14 to 28	IV or IM
	Penicillin G	300,000 units/kg/day	6 divided doses	20 million units/day	14 to 28	IV

Information derived from AAP Red Book[1]

SECTION V

ATYPICAL PNEUMONIA

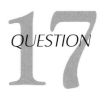

Can You Make a Diagnosis of Atypical Pneumonia by Clinical Presentation or Is Laboratory Evaluation Required?

Christopher R. Cannavino, MD

Atypical pneumonia accounts for a significant proportion of community-acquired pneumonia (CAP) in the pediatric population. There are a number of clinical features that suggest the diagnosis of atypical pneumonia. Although none of these features are pathoneumonic, when taken together, the diagnosis can often be made on clinical presentation alone. Radiographic and laboratory analysis may be useful in certain situations in which the diagnosis is in question. However, routine analysis is not necessary in most children and most commercially available diagnostic tests lack a high level of sensitivity and specificity to reliably distinguish between the causes of CAP. Further, the paucity of clinically useful rapid diagnostic tests for specific atypical pneumonia-associated pathogens limits the utility of such testing. Therefore, a detailed history and physical examination, combined with an understanding of the clinical manifestations and epidemiology of the associated etiologic agents, is fundamental to making a clinical diagnosis of atypical pneumonia.

In 1938, a case series in *JAMA* described acute infection of the respiratory tract with "atypical pneumonia." The patients in the series presented with clinical symptoms differing from those with "typical" pneumococcal pneumonia. Over 60 years later, these differences are still relevant to making a clinical diagnosis of atypical pneumonia. Typical pneumonia, such as that caused by *Streptococcus pneumoniae*, commonly has an abrupt onset of disease with fever, productive cough, and prominent signs of pulmonary consolidation. In contrast, atypical pneumonia commonly has a gradual onset with low-grade fever, dry cough, and less significant symptoms of pulmonary involvement. Further, extrapulmonary symptoms (eg, malaise, upper respiratory tract symptoms, gastrointestinal symptoms) are frequently seen early in the course of an atypical pneumonia prior to the development of respiratory symptoms. These associated symptoms are attributable to the causative pathogen and may give a clue to the etiologic agent, particularly if the clinical presentation fits with the epidemiology of the organism. On physical examination, patients with atypical pneumonia often have diffuse crackles in contrast to the more focal lobar findings commonly seen in typical pneumonia. Wheezing may also be present in some children. The degree of illness is often less than one would expect given the findings on pulmonary examination, leading to the moniker "walking pneumonia." Taken together, these clinical characteristics may distinguish an atypical pneumonia from a pneumonia caused by other bacterial pathogens.

In addition to distinguishing clinical signs and symptoms, epidemiologic clues may aid in the diagnosis of atypical pneumonia. Historically, the most common pathogen associated with atypical pneumonia was *Mycoplasma pneumoniae*, which has long been recognized in adolescents and young adults. More recently, *Chlamydophila pneumoniae* has been described in children and adults (distinct from *Chlamydia trachomatis*, which causes atypical pneumonia in infants). Each pathogen has its own unique epidemiology. *C trachomatis* causes an afebrile pneumonia syndrome in young infants (2 to 19 weeks of age) born to infected mothers. *C pneumoniae* infections are more common in later infancy, preschool-aged, and school-aged children. *M pneumoniae* is most common in school-aged children and adolescents. One study found that children younger than 5 years had lower rates of *M pneumoniae* infections compared with children older than 5 years (15% versus 42%, respectively). Epidemics of *M pneumoniae* infection tend to occur in 4- to 7-year cycles and begin in the fall season. The pattern of illness in the family is occasionally a useful ancillary clue to the causative agent. For instance, in *M pneumoniae*, there are high rates of secondary infection within households, with 2 to 4 weeks elapsing between cases. This pattern is rarely seen in typical bacterial pneumonia.

Routine chest radiographs and laboratory analysis are not necessary for the diagnosis of atypical pneumonia in the outpatient population. Further, such analysis cannot reliably distinguish between atypical and typical CAP. The classic radiographic finding in atypical pneumonia is bilateral patchy, reticulonodular infiltrates with a predilection for the lower lobes. Radiographic findings may suggest a more severe pneumonia than expected based on clinical findings. In comparison, the classic radiographic finding in typical bacterial pneumonia is a unilateral segmental or lobar consolidation. However, studies have shown that chest radiographs lack the proper sensitivity and specificity to differentiate atypical from typical CAP, with lobar and bronchopneumonia occasionally present in children with a reliable diagnosis of *M pneumoniae* infection, and patchy bilateral infiltrates present in children with viral pneumonias. Although the white blood cell count, erythrocyte sedimentation rate, and C-reactive protein tend to be significantly higher in children with typical bacterial pneumonia, the degree of elevation does not reliably distinguish typical from atypical pneumonia and there is considerable overlap between the 2 groups.

For the common etiologic agents of atypical pneumonia, the lack of clinically useful and commercially available diagnostic testing limits the utility of routine testing. Blood cultures do not detect the most common pathogens associated with atypical pneumonia. Thus, the diagnosis must be inferred from serologic testing or detection of the pathogen in the upper respiratory tract. In young infants born to infected mothers, *C trachomatis* is a familiar pathogen of atypical pneumonia. A serum titer of *C trachomatis*–specific immunoglobulin M (IgM) of greater than or equal to 1:32 is considered diagnostic. However, determination of serum antibody concentrations is not available in most clinical laboratories. Culture of respiratory tract secretions, along with associated epithelial cells should be undertaken to attempt confirmation if this diagnosis is suspected, as there are clinical implications for the mother and possibly the father as well. *C pneumoniae*, in contrast, is a common cause of atypical pneumonia in later infancy and school-aged children. However, diagnostic testing for identification of *C pneumoniae* is not reliable, and there is no test for this approved by the US Food and Drug Administration. Serologic testing is most commonly used and an IgM titer of 16 or greater is indicative of acute infection. An immunoglobulin G titer with a 4-fold rise between acute and convalescent serum also indicates acute or recent infection. A single elevated IgG titer should not be used for diagnoses.

M pneumoniae is the most common pathogen associated with atypical pneumonia in school-aged children and adolescents. Diagnostic testing for *M pneumoniae* is commercially available; however, there are a number of factors that limit its clinical utility. Cold agglutination testing lacks the desired sensitivity and specificity. PCR-based testing is available at reference laboratories, but is not useful in an office setting. Serologic assays, including rapid IgM, are widely available and results are often available in a clinically relevant time frame. However, IgM antibodies are generally not present in the first week of illness and may persist for months after an acute infection. Thus, testing is most useful in children with a compatible clinical syndrome in whom there is a high suspicion for *M pneumoniae* but the clinical presentation is not classical. In these select situations, the pretest probability is high and the results yield relatively high sensitivity and specificity and may be used to guide treatment. As a whole, testing for specific pathogens associated with atypical pneumonia lacks clinical utility and is not necessary for routine diagnosis.

So it is possible to make the diagnosis of atypical pneumonia on the basis of clinical presentation alone. The course of illness and presenting signs and symptoms in conjunction with a familiarity with the epidemiology and natural history of the associated pathogens can guide diagnosis and management. In most cases, laboratory testing is not warranted. Although not all patients will present in the classic fashion, the school-aged child with a 1-week history of malaise, sore throat, and low-grade fever who presents with a nonproductive cough and has bilateral crackles and wheezes on pulmonary examination likely has *Mycoplasma* atypical pneumonia and can be treated empirically without laboratory evaluation.

Suggested Readings

Bradley JS, Byington CL, Shah SS, et al. Executive summary: the management of community-acquired pneumonia in infants and children older than 3 months of age: clinical practice guidelines by the Pediatric Infectious Diseases Society and the Infectious Diseases Society of America. *Clin Infect Dis*. 2011;53(7):617-630.

Esposito S, Bosis S, Cavagna R, et al. Characteristics of *Streptococcus pneumoniae* and atypical bacterial infections in children 2-5 years of age with community-acquired pneumonia. *Clin Infect Dis*. 2002;35(11):1345-1352.

Harris JA, Kolokathis A, Cambell M, Cassell GH, Mammerschlag MR. Safety and efficacy of azithromycin in the treatment of community-acquired pneumonia in children. *Pediatr Infect Dis J*. 1998;17(10):865-871.

Michelow IC, Olsen K, Lozano J, et al. Epidemiology and clinical characteristics of community-acquired pneumonia in hospitalized children. *Pediatrics*. 2004;113(4):701-707.

Plouffe JF. Importance of atypical pathogens of community-acquired pneumonia. *Clin Infect Dis*. 2000;31(suppl 2): S35-S39.

Reiman HA. An acute infection of the respiratory tract with atypical pneumonia. *JAMA*. 1938;111(26):2377-2384.

Wubbel L, Muniz L, Ahmed A, et al. Etiology and treatment of community-acquired pneumonia in ambulatory children. *Pediatr Infect Dis J*. 1999;18(2):98-104.

WHAT ARE THE MOST COMMON AGES, PRESENTING SYMPTOMS, AND COMMON ORGANISMS ASSOCIATED WITH CASES OF ATYPICAL PNEUMONIA?

Christopher R. Cannavino, MD

Atypical pneumonia can occur at any age in the pediatric population and accounts for a significant percentage of community-acquired pneumonia (CAP). However, there are classic epidemiologic clues and presenting symptoms that help distinguish atypical pneumonias from other causes of CAP. In general, atypical pneumonia is more common in school-aged children and adolescents. Atypical pneumonias often have a subacute onset and an insidious course. They frequently begin with nonspecific extrapulmonary symptoms, progress to have predominantly lower respiratory tract symptoms, and end with protracted cough. The degree of illness during the lower respiratory tract phase is often less than one would expect given the findings on pulmonary examination. This clinical course characterizes the atypical pneumonias and has led to the colloquialism "walking pneumonia." Atypical pneumonias are caused by a set of unique organisms and the typical age of infection, presenting symptoms, and disease course vary by pathogen.

During early infancy, *Chlamydia trachomatis* is the most common pathogen associated with atypical pneumonia. *C trachomatis* is an obligate intracellular, gram-negative bacterium. It is the most common cause of reportable sexually transmitted infection in the United States. Acquisition of the pathogen occurs in approximately 50% of infants born to infected mothers and, of these, 5% to 20% will develop pneumonia. Infection typically occurs in these young infants between 2 and 19 weeks of age (on average at 6 weeks of age). Affected infants are usually afebrile and otherwise well appearing, leading to afebrile pneumonia syndrome of infancy. *C trachomatis* pneumonia presents insidiously with symptoms gradually worsening over 1 week or more. The classic symptoms consist of tachypnea, rales, and a repetitive staccato cough. Wheezing is rare. Associated symptoms may include nasal congestion and otitis media. Conjunctivitis or a history of neonatal conjunctivitis is present in approximately 50% of affected infants. Hyperinflation and bilateral alveolar and interstitial infiltrates may be present on chest radiographs. Peripheral eosinophilia is a variable finding. When *C trachomatis* pneumonia is suspected, a naso-pharyngeal specimen should be collected for *Chlamydia* culture. Nonculture methods, such as direct fluorescent antibody testing or nucleic acid amplification tests can also be sent, although sensitivity and specificity of nasopharyngeal specimens is lower than with testing of ocular specimens. Notably, direct fluorescent antibody testing is the only Food and Drug Administration (FDA) cleared nonculture test for detection of *C trachomatis* in nasopharyngeal samples. Because test results may not be available promptly, treatment for *C trachomatis* pneumonia is often initiated based on clinical and radiographic findings.

Infants born to mothers with untreated *Chlamydia* infection are at risk for the development of pneumonia and should be monitored closely to ensure appropriate treatment should infection develop. Routine prophylaxis is not recommended, as efficacy of this approach has not been established. Chlamydial conjunctivitis should be treated with systemic rather than topical therapy, to prevent an associated pneumonia.

In later infancy and school-aged children *Chlamydophila* (formerly *Chlamydia*) *pneumoniae* is a common cause of atypical pneumonia. *C pneumoniae* is an obligate intracellular, gram-negative bacterium that is transmitted via respiratory tract secretions. It was previously referred to as the Taiwan acute respiratory (TWAR) agent. Past studies have suggested a median age of approximately 3 years for *C pneumonia*. However, serologic evidence indicates that initial *C pneumoniae* infections are most common between 5 and 15 years of age with a peak in school-aged children 5 to 9 years of age. Definition of the exact epidemiology of *C pneumoniae* is hindered by the lack of well-standardized diagnostic testing. Further, coinfection with other organisms is frequently present and recurrent infection is common. *C pneumoniae* pneumonia typically has a subacute onset followed by a protracted cough lasting 2 to 6 weeks. Upper respiratory tract symptoms may precede the onset of lower respiratory tract symptoms by 1 to 4 weeks, resulting in a biphasic illness. Nonexudative pharyngitis and hoarse voice are common manifestations of the upper respiratory tract phase of illness. The classic lower respiratory tract symptoms consist of rales, rhonchi, and bronchospasm. The cough is typically prominent, nonproductive, and may persist for weeks to months despite appropriate antibiotic therapy. Fever is more common at the onset of illness and may be absent by the time the illness progresses to involve the lower respiratory tract. Associated symptoms may include headache, laryngitis, otitis media, or sinusitis. Chest radiographs typically reveal nonfocal infiltrates. The diagnosis is usually made clinically and macrolides are the empiric treatment of choice.

In school-aged children and adolescents, *Mycoplasma pneumoniae* is the most common cause of atypical pneumonia. *M pneumoniae* is a pleomorphic bacterium that lacks a cell wall and is one of the smallest free-living organisms. Transmission occurs via respiratory droplets. It was first identified as the etiologic agent of primary atypical pneumonia, defined as pneumonia not responsive to antipneumococcal therapy, and was previously referred to as *Eaton agent*. Although *M pneumoniae* is a frequent cause of atypical pneumonia in older children, it is less commonly implicated in children younger than 5 years. Newer studies show that *Mycoplasma* may be an underrecognized pathogen in preschool-aged children; however, there appears to be a high rate of clinical resolution irrespective of effective antimycoplasma treatment. The secondary attack rate in households is approximately 40%, although transmission is slow, with intervals of 2 to 3 weeks between cases. There is typically a gradual progression of symptoms with initial malaise, head-ache, sore throat, and low-grade fever giving way to lower respiratory tract symptoms over 3 to 5 days. Clinical signs and symptoms of atypical pneumonia include diffuse crackles and cough. In fact, cough is the hallmark of pneumonia caused by *Mycoplasma*; it is initially nonproductive, is typically the reason children seek medical care and may, despite treatment, last for weeks after the resolution of other symptoms. *M pneumoniae* is commonly associated with wheezing and asthma exacerbations may occur in children with atopy. The findings on physical examination are often disproportionate to the degree of illness. Associated symptoms may include pharyngitis, otitis media, and myringitis. A maculopapular rash may accompany the pneumonia in up to 10% of children. Unusual manifestations, including central nervous system disease such as meningoencephalitis, may be associated with *Mycoplasma* infections. Chest radiographs most commonly show bilateral, diffuse infiltrates, although focal abnormalities may occur. Diagnosis is typically made clinically, although laboratory testing is available. As *M pneumoniae* lacks a cell wall, the beta-lactam antibiotics are ineffective. Treatment is similar to that for *C pneumoniae*.

There are other pathogens associated with atypical pneumonia; however, they are rare in the pediatric population. For these uncommon causes, there is often an exposure history that aids in the diagnosis. For instance, psittacosis (*Chlamydia psittaci*), Q fever (*Coxiella burnetii*), and tularemia (*Francisella tularensis*) all may manifest as an atypical pneumonia in the setting of a child with zoonotic exposures (birds, sheep/domestic farm animals, and rabbits/wild mammals, respectively). Although *Legionella* is an important cause of atypical pneumonia in adults, it is only rarely seen in children and is associated with milder clinical manifestations.

Thus, atypical pneumonia is a relatively common diagnosis in the pediatric population. Atypical pneumonia usually has a subacute presentation and indolent course. Most children present with cough and lower respiratory tract symptoms and have a history of preceding extrapulmonary symptoms. The most common pathogens are *C pneumoniae* in older infants and school-aged children and *M pneumoniae* in school-aged children and adolescents. A familiarity with the epidemiology and clinical manifestations of atypical pneumonia may aid in the diagnosis and guide treatment in children with CAP.

Suggested Readings

Aldous MB, Grayston JT, Wang SP, Foy HM. Seroepidemiology of *Chlamydia pneumoniae* TWAR infection in Seattle families, 1966–1979. *J Infect Dis.* 1992;166(3):646-649.

American Academy of Pediatrics. Chlamydial infections. In: Pickering LK, Baker CJ, Kimberlin DW, Long SS, eds. *Red Book: 2009 Report of the Committee on Infectious Diseases.* 28th ed. Elk Grove Village, IL: American Academy of Pediatrics; 2009:252-259.

American Academy of Pediatrics. *Mycoplasma pneumoniae* and other *Mycoplasma* species infections. In: Pickering LK, Baker CJ, Kimberlin DW, Long SS, eds. *Red Book: 2009 Report of the Committee on Infectious Diseases.* 28th ed. Elk Grove Village, IL: American Academy of Pediatrics; 2009:473-475.

Bradley JS, Byington CL, Shah SS, et al. Executive summary: the management of community-acquired pneumonia in infants and children older than 3 months of age: clinical practice guidelines by the Pediatric Infectious Diseases Society and the Infectious Diseases Society of America. *Clin Infect Dis.* 2011;53(7):617-630.

Burillo A, Bouza E. *Chlamydophila pneumoniae. Infect Dis Clin North Am.* 2010;24(1):61-71.

Centers for Disease Control and Prevention. Sexually transmitted diseases treatment guidelines, 2010. *MMWR.* 2010;59(No. RR-12):47-48.

Michelow IC, Olsen K, Lozano J, et al. Epidemiology and clinical characteristics of community-acquired pneumonia in hospitalized children. *Pediatrics.* 2004;113(4):701-707.

Tipple MA, Beem MO, Saxon EM. Clinical characteristics of the afebrile pneumonia associated with *Chlamydia trachomatis* infection in infants less than 6 months of age. *Pediatrics.* 1979;63(2):192-197.

SECTION VI

OTITIS MEDIA

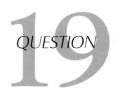

WHAT IS THE RECOMMENDED SPECIFIC TREATMENT OF OTITIS MEDIA DUE TO MULTIDRUG-RESISTANT PNEUMOCOCCUS?

Christopher J. Harrison, MD

New data published in *The New England Journal of Medicine* in January 2011 showed benefits of antibiotic treatment for acute otitis media (AOM) in children 6 to 36 months of age. Therefore, treatment of symptomatic AOM in young children is acceptable based on the evidence.[1] The last rigorous set of guidelines was released by the American Academy of Pediatrics (AAP) in 2005 and is currently being revised. The guidelines mainly target 2 specific pathogens, *Streptococcus pneumoniae* (SP) and nontypeable *Haemophilus influenzae* (ntHi). To get a better picture of the likely pathogens in intermittent AOM (no episodes in prior 30 days) versus persistent or recurrent AOM, see Figure 19-1. Amoxicillin-resistant pathogens (penicillin nonsusceptible SP [PNSP] or beta-lactamase-producing ntHi) are more likely in recurrent or persistent AOM mostly due to recent antibiotic exposure.

What do practitioners need to know about recent and expected changes in AOM related to pneumococcus given the long-standing use of 7-valent pneumococcal conjugate vaccine (PCV7) and the 2010 release of PCV13? Based on data from the PCV7 era in 2000–2010, ntHi (particularly beta-lactamase-producing strains) became the most frequent AOM pathogen among children adequately immunized with PCV7. However, SP (mostly nonvaccine types) remained nearly as common, but the serotypes causing AOM had changed. Serotype 19A, which is now included in PCV13, emerged as the most common single SP serotype, whereas the previous amoxicillin-resistant PCV7 types nearly disappeared. To make matters more difficult, the emerging 19A strains were often even more resistant (multidrug-resistant [MDR]). Further, MDR 19A strains commonly show high levels of resistance to clindamycin, azithromycin, all oral cephalosporins, and trimethoprim sulfamethoxazole.[2] So how does one choose an antibiotic for AOM (Table 19-1)?

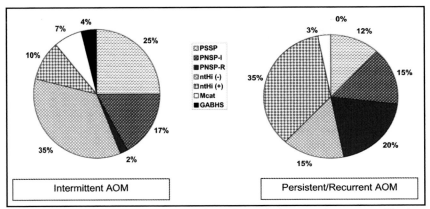

Figure 19-1. GABHS = group A beta-hemolytic streptococcus; Mcat = *M catarrhalis*; ntHi = nontypebale H influenzae; PSSP = penicillin-susceptible *S pneumoniae*; PNSP-I = penicillin nonsusceptible *S pneumoniae*–intermediate resistance; PNSP-R = penicillin-nonsusceptible *S pneumoniae*–highly resistant; (–) = beta-lactamase negative; (+) = beta-lactamase positive.[3]

Table 19-1

Drugs of Choice for Acute Otitis Media

		PCN Nonallergic	*PCN Allergy— Mild to Moderate*	*PCN Allergy— Severe*
Intermittent AOM	First line	Amoxicillin HD	Cefdinir HD	Clindamycin + TMP/S
Persistent/recurrent AOM	Second line	Amoxicillin + Clavulanate HD	Clindamycin + cefixime (or cefdinir)	Clindamycin + Tmp/S
AOM failing second-line therapy	Third line	Ceftriaxone IM	Levofloxacin*	Levofloxacin*

*Not FDA approved for AOM but data are published on efficacy. See p. 100 AAP 2009 edition of Red Book for quinolone statements.

Intermittent Acute Otitis Media

NO ALLERGY TO PENICILLIN

The drug of choice remains high-dose amoxicillin (90 mg/kg/d divided into 2 doses), which covers ~80% of 19A strains and nearly 100% of other SP. The weakness is that beta-lactamase-producing ntHi (making up ~15% of intermittent AOM and 45% of recurrent AOM) are resistant to any dose of amoxicillin. So high-dose amoxicillin covers ~85% of intermittent AOM.

Nonsevere Amoxicillin Allergy or Intolerance

For nonanaphylactic allergy to amoxicillin, oral cephalosporins might seem to be reasonable choices. However, 2010 data from our laboratory indicate that 50% of SP are resistant to all oral cephalosporins including cefuroxime axetil, cefpodoxime proxetil, and cefdinir, even high-dose cefdinir (25 to 30 mg/kg/d). Furthermore, 100% of MDR SP are resistant to every oral cephalosporin. Therefore, those failing high-dose amoxicillin should expect little benefit against SP from oral cephalosporins. Their benefit is greater for ntHi (beta-lactamase producing and nonproducing), with 80% being susceptible to cefdinir and more than 95% susceptible to either cefuroxime axetil or cefpodoxime proxetil. Cefdinir tastes better but is likely to produce ~10% fewer cures. So for intermittent AOM, oral cephalosporins could be used but failures should be expected for ~80% SP and 20% ntHi. Azithromycin also might seem reasonable in this scenario, but it is not acceptable for almost any AOM episode. Further data from our laboratory show that nearly 100% of ntHi are resistant to azithromycin and 30% to 50% of SP are also resistant to azithromycin. Failures should be expected in half of ntHi AOM episodes (50% spontaneously resolve; otherwise, there would be 100% failures with ntHi) and ~40% of SP episodes. Therefore, azithromycin is a poor choice to treat even intermittent AOM given current data.

Severe Amoxicillin Allergy

In this situation, oral cephalosporins are not attractive options. Use of clindamycin at 30 mg/kg/d divided in 3 doses for SP plus trimethoprim sulfamethoxazole (10 mg/kg/d of trimethoprim component divided twice daily) for ntHi is an option. This would be expected to cover 90% of SP and 80% to 85% of ntHi. Consider using a preemptive probiotic with this combination.

Recurrent/Persistent Acute Otitis Media

No Penicillin Allergy

High-dose amoxicillin-clavulanate is the best choice. This covers not only the large majority of SP, including 80% of serotype 19A, but also more than 95% of beta-lactamase-producing ntHi. This provides activity against 85% of the early treatment failures while on amoxicillin and ~80% to 90% of recurrent AOM (prior episode in last 30 days). So a strategy for AOM involving the sequence of amoxicillin followed by amoxicillin-clavulanate, due to initial amoxicillin failure, predicts more than 95% overall cure rate.

Nonsevere Amoxicillin Allergy
or Amoxicillin–Clavulanate Intolerance

The problems noted for alternative drugs in the discussion about first-line AOM drugs persist but are amplified when considering second-line AOM therapy given that a cephalosporin was used as the first-line drug. In this situation, a high proportion are MDR SP. So no oral cephalosporin alone is likely to have more than 20% efficacy against SP that survive the initial oral cephalosporin. One option is to combine clindamycin (80% to 85% SP coverage) with a potent anti-ntHi cephalosporin such as cefixime (98% ntHi coverage). Alternatively, a 3-dose ceftriaxone strategy could be useful here. My suggestion is to give a dose on day 1 and repeat a dose every other day for a maximum of 3 doses, but repeat doses only if the child continues to have symptoms. This will result in roughly a third of patients getting 1, 2, or 3 doses, respectively.

TRUE SEVERE PENICILLIN ALLERGY OR DRUG INTOLERANCE

Clindamycin that would cover 60% to 80% MDR SP is an alternative, but to provide empiric coverage for ntHi, trimethoprim sulfamethoxazole would be necessary. This combination might be expected to have a higher rate of gastrointestinal side effects than even amoxicillin plus clavulanate, so again consider a preemptive probiotic.

Third-Line Acute Otitis Media Drug

NO PENICILLIN ALLERGY

For failures of sequential amoxicillin and amoxicillin-clavulanate, intramuscular ceftri-axone doses of 50 mg/kg/d for 3 days as noted above is recommended, expecting this to cure 90% of the few subjects failing the sequential oral strategy.

TRUE SEVERE PENICILLIN ALLERGY OR DRUG INTOLERANCE

Some practitioners dislike 3 once-daily doses of injectable antibiotic. In these cases or with concern for a true cephalosporin allergy, creative choices are needed. They are not Food and Drug Administration (FDA) approved for children with AOM, and it is necessary to inform families as such. Levofloxacin covers 99% of SP and 100% of ntHi. The hip dysplasia or cartilage damage concerns based on animal studies have not been confirmed and the American Academy of Pediatrics Committee on Infectious Diseases' *Red Book* indicates that quinolone use is reasonable when there is no alternative, particularly among oral drugs.[4] Linezolid plus trimethoprim sulfamethoxazole is another possible choice, but linezolid is the most expensive oral antibiotic and can cause suppression of bone marrow if used for more than 2 weeks.

Which types of SP currently have the most drug resistance? If we look at this in terms of strains included in PCV13 or those in neither PCV vaccine, a pattern seems to be developing. Half of the drug-resistant SP isolated from upper respiratory tract cultures are represented in PCV13, but half are not.

Among those not in PCV13, some have intermediate resistance to penicillin. Among these, resistance is found in 100% to azithromycin, 75% to oral cephalosporins, 12% to clindamycin, and 0% to ceftriaxone. Those strains not in PCV13 but with high-level resistance to penicillin have resistance in 85% to azithromycin, 90% to oral cephalosporins, 40% to clindamycin, and 20% to ceftriaxone. Of the 73 MDR-SP isolates from the Kansas City area that were tested from 2007 to 2010, none were found to be resistant to levofloxacin or linezolid.

Even if PCV13 completely eliminates all serotypes contained within it, including serotype 19A, it appears that multidrug resistance will remain with us; and the oral cephalosporins as well as azithromycin will remain poor choices for those who fail initial therapy with high-dose amoxicillin.

References

1. Klein JO. Is acute otitis media a treatable disease? *N Engl J Med.* 2011;364(2):168-169.
2. Harrison CJ, Woods C, Stout GG, Martin B, Selvarangan R. Susceptibilities of *Haemophilus influenzae*, *Streptococcus pneumoniae*, including serotype 19A, and *Moraxella catarrhalis* pediatric isolates from 2005-2007 to commonly used antibiotics. *J Antimicrob Chemother.* 2009(3);63:511-519.
3. Harrison CJ. The changing microbiology of acute otitis media. In: *Acute Otitis Media: Translating Science Into Clinical Practice, International Congress and Symposium Series* 265. London: Royal Society of Medicine Press; 2007:22-35.
4. American Academy of Pediatrics. Lyme disease. In: Pickering LK, Baker CJ, Kimberlin DW, Long SS, eds. *Red Book: 2009 Report of the Committee on Infectious Diseases.* 28th ed. Elk Grove Village, IL: American Academy of Pediatrics; 2009:430-435.

Suggested Readings

Harrison CJ. The microbiology of AOM: past, present, and future. *Suppl Contemporary Pediatr,* 2005;22(12):8-16.
Shaikh N, Hoberman A, Kearney DH, Yellon R. Videos in clinical medicine. Tympanocentesis in children with acute otitis media. *N Engl J Med.* 2011;364(2):e4.

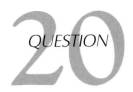

WHEN SHOULD MIDDLE EAR EFFUSION FLUID BE OBTAINED?

Christopher J. Harrison, MD

Tympanocentesis was a standard treatment for relief of acute otitis media (AOM)–related pain before the availability of antibiotics. Although the act of puncturing the tympanic membrane (TM) may sound scary and difficult to perform, the short (<10 seconds during the procedure and shortly after the actual puncture) amount of pain are of true benefit to the patient, and it is less difficult to perform than a lumbar puncture or radial artery puncture. It requires minimum equipment (lance or suction apparatus), isopropyl alcohol, topical anesthetic, firm restraint of the patient, and culture media.[1] There are up to 3 days of mild otorrhea thereafter, but no serious sequelae should occur. Despite this, the relatively simple procedure became unnecessary after 1965 when antibiotics cured nearly 95% of cases. So why did the CDC Drug-Resistant *Streptococcus pneumoniae* Therapeutic Working Group and the 2004 American Academy of Pediatrics (AAP)/American Academy of Family Practice (AAFP) guidelines for managing uncomplicated AOM recommend this procedure?[2]

It was because increasing clinical failures were noted in the 1990s and early in the new millennium, mostly due to multidrug-resistant *Streptococcus pneumoniae* (MDR-SP) and beta-lactamase–producing nontypeable *Haemophilus influenzae* (ntHi).[3] From 1995 to 2002, most otitis media infections (~70%) continued to be caused by susceptible pneumococcus or susceptible ntHi. However, MDR-SP infections were mostly caused by serotypes that ultimately were included in the 7-valent pneumococcal conjugate vaccine (PCV7), which was released in 2000. These serotypes are 6B, 9V, 14, 19F, and 23F. By 2004, nearly all MDR-SP had become non-PCV7 strains and type 19A had become the biggest problem.

In fact, MDR 19A strains had become uniformly resistant to all oral cephalosporins and trimethoprim-sulfamethoxazole, highly resistant to azithromycin, ~70% resistant to clindamycin, and resistant to standard dosing of amoxicillin. The most effective outpatient therapy now is limited to high-dose amoxicillin (90 to 100 mg/kg/d divided into 2 doses) with resistance noted in ~20% MDR-SP and 30% ntHi. Alternative options include 3 single daily 50 mg/kg IM doses of ceftriaxone (resistance in ~15% MDR-SP but none in ntHi) or 10 mg/kg twice daily doses of levofloxacin (resistance in <2% MDR-SP and none in ntHi).

This increased clinical failure rate resulted in the AAP and AAFP recommending tympanocentesis for clinical failures after either a third consecutive antibiotic course or ceftriaxone for 3 days.

The rationale was that tympanocentesis with culture removes the majority of the infecting bacterial load, relieves accompanying pressure-related otalgia, and allows pathogen-specific antibiotic choice. However, few clinicians have been trained to perform tympanocentesis.[4] So, most cases that need tympanocentesis must be referred to an experienced practitioner of the art. Workshops were sponsored by the AAP to teach this skill, but the idea never really caught on.

Why is there less call for tympanocentesis since 2006? It seems that despite the emergence of 19A MDR-SP, the absolute numbers of AOM persisting despite either 3 consecutive antibiotic courses or after ceftriaxone for 3 days had decreased as had the total numbers of AOM overall. This has been attributed to both the effects of PCV7[5,6] and education on more strict criteria for diagnosis of AOM. Some practitioners also began using levofloxacin. The demand for treatment of recalcitrant AOM had decreased.

What may reduce the need even further was the release in mid-2010 of PCV13, which contains serotype 19A among 5 other added serotypes. This likely will reduce the MDR-SP prevalence dramatically over the next few years. There are some data suggesting that types 27, 33, and 35 may be emerging as we reduce 19A prevalence, but only type 35 shows notable antibiotic resistance as of the beginning of 2011.

Having said that, there will still be cases that need tympanocentesis. These cases will be the same but lesser numbers of recalcitrant AOM patients as noted above, plus AOM in immune-compromised hosts where pseudomonas, MDR gram-negative organisms, or even methicillin-resistant *Staphylococcus aureus* are more likely pathogens. In these cases, culture of middle ear effusion (MEE) can be the key to appropriate antimicrobial choices.

In all cases, tympanocentesis should only be performed when AOM (purulent or infected MEE) is assured. The AAP/AAFP 2004 guidelines' criteria for AOM are too inclusive.[2] These guidelines allow any type of MEE (even that of otitis media with effusion [OME]) with a distinctly red (TM) plus other symptoms to be considered AOM. The approach to diagnosis of AOM should require an inflamed, opaque, and bulging TM to meet criteria. Otherwise a "dry tap" may occur or one may obtain a sterile noninfected effusion from OME that happens to occur in a febrile child. Remember that diffuse erythema of the TM can occur with crying in an infant, or more focally as hypervascularity, particularly near the annulus and visible ossicles on the TM in OME or as part of the natural residual up to 2 weeks after successfully treating AOM.

The rate for pathogen recovery from tympanocentesis depends only on tapping true AOM cases and meticulous handling of the procedure and specimen. Highest yields (up to 90%) occur with immediate inoculation onto culture media. Recovery of pathogens after antibiotics is less than 50%. The bacterial detection rate will be suboptimal if residual isopropyl alcohol used to sterilize the external canal or the topical anesthetic is not thoroughly removed.

Most experienced tympanocentesis practitioners report no serious complications. I have not observed any in over 1000 procedures. Temporary (<30 seconds) vertigo occurs in some children old enough to report it. Possible published adverse effects include chronic TM perforation (much less risk than with a tympanostomy tube), bleeding from accidentally piercing the posterior middle ear wall and the internal bulb of the jugular vein (occurs only if the needle is inserted too deep), piercing the oval window (this should not occur with puncture of the proper TM site), disruption of the ossicles with possible hearing loss (also should not occur if proper site punctured), or permanent hearing loss (only occurs with ossicle disruption, which should not occur with proper technique).

References

1. Block SL. Tympanocentesis: why, when, how. *Contemporary Pediatr.* 1999;16:103-127.
2. American Academy of Pediatrics Subcommittee on Management of Acute Otitis Media. Diagnosis and management of acute otitis media. *Pediatrics.* 2004;113(5):1451-1465.
3. Dowell SF, Butler JC, Giebink GS, et al. Acute otitis media: management and surveillance in an era of pneumococcal resistance—a report from the Drug-resistant *Streptococcus pneumoniae* Therapeutic Working Group. *Pediatr Infect Dis J.* 1999;18(1):1-9.
4. Vayalumkal J, Kellner JD. Tympanocentesis for the management of acute otitis media in children. A survey of Canadian pediatricians and family physicians. *Arch Pediatr Adolesc Med.* 2004;158(10):962-965.
5. Harrison CJ, Woods C, Stout GS, Martin B, Selavarangen R. Susceptibilities of *Haemophilus influenzae*, *Streptococcus pneumoniae*, including serotype 19A, and *Moraxella catarrhalis* pediatric isolates from 2005-2007 to commonly used antibiotics. *J Antimicrob Chemother.* 2009;63(3):511-519. doi: 10.1093/jac/dkn538.
6. Casey JR, Adlowitz DG, Pichichero ME. New patterns in the otopathogens causing acute otitis media six to eight years after introduction of pneumococcal conjugate vaccine. *Pediatr Infect Dis J.* 2010;29:304-309.

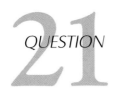

WHAT DO YOU DO FOR A PATIENT WHO HAS EAR TUBES AND HAS CONTINUOUS EAR DRAINAGE?

Christopher J. Harrison, MD

Over half a million children undergo placement of tympanostomy tubes annually. Many will develop otorrhea in the first weeks after placement and this is not unexpected. Most of these respond to conservative or even topical therapy. The problem arises when a child develops frequently recurrent or persisting otorrhea. This can be challenging and often requires collaboration between the primary care provider and the otolaryngologist and may result in frequent visits to both providers that can often be frustrating to parents and providers alike. There are guidelines from selected groups on treating otorrhea; a recent one from Canada is particularly useful.[1]

Intermittent Otorrhea

For those with intermittent otorrhea, pathogens that are isolated by careful culture obtained within 24 hours of the onset of otorrhea and from the lumen of the pressure-equalizing (PE) tube are the same as the spectrum and proportions detected from acute otitis media (AOM) without the presence of PE tubes. These include *Streptococcus pneumoniae*, nontypeable *Haemophilus influenzae*, *Moraxella catarrhalis*, and the occasional group A streptococcus. Treatment of these can usually be undertaken with a topical quinolone such as ciprofloxacin or ofloxacin. Resolution rates occur in 70% to 80% with this therapy.[2] Those failing to respond to topical therapy usually respond to the same oral antibiotics as those prescribed for nondraining AOM. See Question 19 regarding intermittent versus persistent/recurrent AOM.

But what does one do when both of these routine approaches fail to resolve the otorrhea or if otorrhea returns rapidly and frequently despite such therapy? These patients require extra consideration about the pathogens that might be causing it.

Cultures

This raises the question about the utility of culturing material draining from children with chronic otorrhea. When considering culture of otorrhea, it is ideal to obtain specimens less than 36 hours after the onset of otorrhea to prevent contamination by external ear canal pathogens such as *Pseudomonas sp*, particularly if the specimen is obtained from the canal itself. With chronic otorrhea or recurrent otorrhea of more than 2 days duration, one can still obtain accurate cultures. However, this requires cleaning the external canal and obtaining the specimen directly from the opening of the PE tube. This usually requires a visit to the otolaryngologist.

Appropriately obtained cultures can be quite helpful in deciding how to treat chronic otorrhea. If the pathogens are those normally seen with AOM as noted above, then therapeutic success is more likely and a combination of topical plus systemic therapy may be more useful than either alone. However, it seems that unusual and multidrug-resistant pathogens are becoming more frequent. These include methicillin-susceptible *Staphylococcus aureus* (MSSA), methicillin-resistant *Staphylococcus aureus* (MRSA), *Pseudomonas aeruginosa*, *Acinetobacter baumanni*, various species of *Candida*, and sometimes even *Aspergillus* species. A common characteristic of these unusual pathogens is their affinity for foreign bodies, including PE tubes.

Aural Toilet

One must have a reasonable expectation when treating these organisms because medical therapy alone may fail as often as half the time. It is good to share this with parents when embarking on a treatment regimen. In the ideal situation, cleaning the external ear canal 2 to 3 times a week helps reduce the inoculum and the inflammatory debris such that success of antimicrobial therapy is enhanced. This can be difficult to schedule both from the family and otolaryngologist standpoints. However, it has been my experience that adding this "aural toilet" to antimicrobial therapy improves the chance of success.

Specific Antimicrobials

When attempting to medically treat chronic otorrhea apparently due to *Staphylococcus aureus*, whether MRSA or MSSA, consider using a 3-week course with a pathogen-specific primary drug based on susceptibilities. For example, for MRSA, clindamycin or trimethoprim sulfamethoxazole may be a primary drug. For MSSA, trimethoprim sulfamethoxazole or a cephalosporin with MSSA activity (cefuroxime axetil, cefpodoxime proxetil, or cefdinir) may act as the primary drug. In either instance, success may be enhanced by the addition of rifampin at 10 mg/kg/d. Remember that cefdinir is the least active of the three cephalosporins against MSSA and should be used at high dose (25 to 30 mg/kg/d). Also note that cephalexin and cefadroxil do not penetrate into the middle ear space and are not recommended as treatment in any form of middle ear infection. As an auxiliary drug, rifampin has been shown to improve success by ~25% when treating staphylococcal infections of prostheses such as those used in joint replacement.[3,4]

Treating *Pseudomonas sp*, *Acinetobacter sp*, or other gram-negative organisms often classified as "water bugs" can be challenging because prior topical therapy often selects for resistance to quinolones. In these situations, resistance as defined by the breakpoints usually utilized in clinical microbiology laboratories for systemic infections may not be entirely predictive of potential success.

Topicals

Topical therapy has the advantage of delivering hundreds of micrograms of drug, concentrations beyond those achievable with oral or even intravenous administration. Colistin is often active even against gram-negative pathogens resistant to standard drugs, but topical preparations approved for use in the external ear also usually contain neomycin (Cortisporin; Pfizer Inc, New York, NY), which can sensitize mucosa and actually add to otorrhea. However, colistin sulfate otic drops can be compounded if you have access to a compounding pharmacy. A combination formulation of a quinolone plus a corticosteroid (Ciprodex; Alcon, Fort Worth, TX) also has been shown to have an advantage over the quinolone alone, particularly if the mucosa of the middle ear has developed a secretory component due to the chronic inflammation.

However, some organisms remain clinically resistant to treatment with any of the standard antimicrobial or even specially compounded topical agents. In such situations a topical antiseptic, such as acetic acid (Vosol Otic; Hi Tech Pharmacal Co. Inc, Amityville, NY), may sometimes provide resolution when antimicrobials do not. Of note, acetic acid can cause a burning sensation on installation and this may limit its utility. There are acetic acid formulations that also include a corticosteroid for suppressing inflammation, so it can still be worth a try to use these topical agents.

It is useful when administering topical drops into the ear canal to first use a wick to remove as much of the debris as possible before adding the drops. If the canal is relatively clear, putting pressure on the tragus to close over the orifice and then pumping up and down 2 to 3 times may aid in delivery of the drops to the infected area.

Caveat

Topical preparations containing antimicrobials and/or corticosteroids can select for fungal pathogens. Even without such selection, frequent oral antibiotics may select for these agents as well. *Candida albicans*, *Candida tropicalis*, and *Candida parapsilosis* are the most frequently identified. These may respond to 2 weeks of a combination of oral fluconazole plus a topical acetic acid preparation. When *Aspergillus* species are found in the middle ear, referral to an otolaryngologist and/or infectious disease specialist is prudent. These are particularly difficult to treat and often require removal of the pressure-equalizing tubes.

Medical Treatment Failures

Despite our best efforts in obtaining accurate cultures, and using susceptibility driven antimicrobials or other topicals, up to 50% can still fail medical therapy even using the longer 3-week courses. At this point, repeating cultures may be helpful because therapy may have selected for a new pathogen. This could allow redirecting therapy. However, often the pathogen is persistent and has become more resistant than the original strain. This requires consultation with the otolaryngologist with the idea that the PE tubes most likely will need to be removed. Hopefully, the child will not develop recurrent middle ear disease that caused placement of the PE tubes in the first place, but if this happens, an interval of several months prior to placement of the new PE tubes is usually warranted.

References

1. Schmelzle J, Birtwhistle RV, Tan AK. Acute otitis media in children with tympanostomy tubes. *Can Fam Physician.* 2008;54(8):1123-1127.
2. Roland PS, Kreisler LS, Reese B, et al. Topical ciprofloxacin/dexamethasone otic suspension is superior to ofloxacin otic solution in the treatment of children with acute otitis media with otorrhea through tympanostomy tubes. *Pediatrics.* 2004;113(1 Pt 1):e40-e46.
3. Forrest GN, Tamura K. Rifampin combination therapy for nonmycobacterial infections. *Clin Microbiol Rev.* 2010;23(1):14-34.
4. Zimmerli W, Widmer AF, Blatter M, Frei R, Ochsner PE. Role of rifampin for treatment of orthopedic implant-related staphylococcal infections: a randomized controlled trial. Foreign-Body Infection (FBI) Study Group. *JAMA.*1998;279(19):1537-1541.

Suggested Readings

Coticchia JM, Dohar JE. Methicillin-resistant *Staphylococcus aureus* otorrhea after tympanostomy tube placement. *Arch Otolaryngol Head Neck Surg.* 2005;131(10):868-873.

Granath A, Rynnel-Dagoo B, Backheden M, Lindberg K. Tube associated otorrhea in children with recurrent acute otitis media; results of a prospective randomized study on bacteriology and topical treatment with or without systemic antibiotics. *Int J Pediatr Otorhinolaryngol.* 2008;72(8):1225-1233.

Heslop A, Lildholdt T, Gammelgaard N, Ovesen T. Topical ciprofloxacin is superior to topical saline and systemic antibiotics in the treatment of tympanostomy tube otorrhea in children: the results of a randomized clinical trial. *Laryngoscope.* 2010;120(12):2516-2520.

Martin TJ, Kerschner JE, Flanary VA. Fungal causes of otitis externa and tympanostomy tube otorrhea. *Int J Pediatr Otorhinolaryngol.* 2005;69(11):1503-1508.

Roland PS, Anon JB, Moe RD, et al. Topical ciprofloxacin/dexamethasone is superior to ciprofloxacin alone in pediatric patients with acute otitis media and otorrhea through tympanostomy tubes. *Laryngoscope.* 2003;113(12):2116-2122.

Ruohola A, Heikkinen T, Meurman O, Puhakka T, Lindblad N, Ruuskanen O. Antibiotic treatment of acute otorrhea through tympanostomy tube: randomized double-blind placebo-controlled study with daily follow-up. *Pediatrics.* 2003;111(5):1061-1067.

WHAT IS THE RECOMMENDED SPECIFIC TREATMENT OF ACUTE OTITIS MEDIA DUE TO MULTIDRUG-RESISTANT PNEUMOCOCCUS?

Christopher J. Harrison, MD

It is uncommon in routine practice for clinicians to have culture results for acute otitis media (AOM). Most of the time, AOM treatment choices are empiric, based on the most likely pathogens for a given patient presentation. For example, children with intermittent AOM (no episodes within the last month) have less than 5% chance to have multidrug-resistant (MDR) pneumococcus. In contrast, patients who have symptomatic AOM persisting beyond 3 to 5 days of initial empiric therapy or those with recurrent AOM at less than 1 month after the last episode have an almost 25% chance to have MDR pneumococcus. Therefore, strategies to treat MDR pneumococcus are often useful when treating persistent or recurrent AOM but are not likely to be needed for intermittent AOM. There are situations in which spontaneous perforation of the tympanic membranes occurs, and this allows the clinician the opportunity to obtain a culture. In addition, children who have pressure-equalizing tubes in place can drain through the tubes, and therefore offer a similar opportunity for culture.

Serotype 19A

When MDR pneumococcus is detected and then is subsequently serotyped, the overwhelming majority is serotype 19A. These strains became dominant since the introduction of heptavalent pneumococcal conjugate vaccine (PCV7). With the introduction of PCV13 in June 2010, there is the expectation that serotype 19A will likely decrease dramatically over the next few years. Whether other MDR strains that are now uncommon, such as serotype 35 and 21, will expand to fill the niche relinquished by serotype 19A remains to be seen.

Definition of Multidrug-Resistant Pneumococcus

When culture results and susceptibilities are available, what is a microbiological definition of MDR pneumococcus? Usually, MDR pneumococcal strains are resistant to penicillin (and by virtue of this they will be resistant to all oral cephalosporins), macrolides, and trimethoprim sulfamethoxazole. Nearly 40% are also resistant to clindamycin but only 20% to 30% are resistant to ceftriaxone. They are uniformly susceptible to linezolid and more than 97% are susceptible to levofloxacin.

With this definition, it is easy to see why treatment of MDR pneumococcus could be a challenge in the outpatient setting where AOM patients present. The simple answer is that one can use the narrowest spectrum oral drug to which the pathogen is susceptible. However, most MDR pneumococcal strains do not offer a simple choice. Most strains are resistant in vitro to most of our usual AOM drugs; however, there are nuances to the resistance to the different drugs that allow some options that do not mandate creative unlabeled use, use of unusual drug combinations, or even parenteral drugs.

Amoxicillin Still Works for Most Multidrug-Resistant Pneumococcus in Acute Otitis Media

There are 2 reasons for this. First, resistance to penicillin is not an absolute phenomenon. This translates to the fact that high-dose amoxicillin will often be successful in treating MDR pneumococcus in the middle ear. Studies using the double tap experimental design, in which patients undergo tympanocentesis just before starting therapy and then have repeat tympanocentesis on approximately day 5 of therapy, have shown that pneumococcal strains with minimum inhibitory concentrations (MICs) of less than or equal to 4.0 mg/L respond to treatment with high-dose amoxicillin at 90 to 100 mg/kg/d divided in 2 doses. Secondly, only 25% of MDR pneumococcus have MICs to amoxicillin of more than 4.0 mg/L (Figure 22-1). Many experts recommend that one initially prescribes high-dose amoxicillin unless there is an anaphylactic-type allergy to penicillin.

This then raises the question as to whether high-dose amoxicillin is still appropriate with recurrent AOM within 30 days of finishing high-dose amoxicillin. A study performed by Leibovitz et al showed that for each consecutive week after finishing therapy, the chances decrease dramatically of having a persistent organism that failed initial therapy. Over 50% are new pathogens even within the first week after finishing previous therapy, but this rises to ~90% new pathogens if AOM recurs in the fourth week after discontinuing prior AOM therapy.[1] So it is unlikely, if one initially responds to amoxicillin, that the pathogen involved in the recurrent AOM is the same strain. What likely causes the recurrent or sometimes even persistent AOM are pathogens that have been selected by the initial therapy. The most likely pathogens selected in this fashion are beta-lactamase–producing nontypeable *Haemophilus influenzae* (ntHi) and somewhat less likely MDR pneumococcus. It is not highly penicillin-resistant MDR pneumococcus that usually

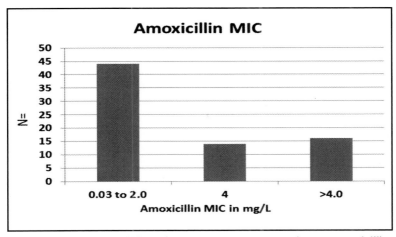

Figure 22-1. Susceptibility of *Streptococcus pneumoniae* to amoxicillin. Efficacy of high-dose amoxicillin expected to be higher than 90% for 0.03 to 2.0 mg/L, 60% for 4.0 mg/L, and 20% for higher than 4.0 mg/L.

requires an alternative to high-dose amoxicillin, but it is the beta-lactamase–producing organisms that make up ~40% of persistent or recurrent AOM.

If we know that MDR pneumococcus is present, the beta-lactamase issue is not relevant. There has never been a pneumococcus that produces beta-lactamase. Pneumococcus is resistant to amoxicillin by virtue of mutated penicillin-binding proteins (PBPs). Beta-lactam drugs can bind to and inactivate most PBPs, even mutated PBPs. However, they must physically bind to the PBP to provide antimicrobial activity.

Native (no mutations) PBPs actively attract beta-lactam drugs like a magnet does iron filings, but when PBPs mutate this attraction decreases proportional to the number and degree of mutation. So instead of amoxicillin molecules being actively pulled toward the bacteria from anywhere nearby, the amoxicillin must by random chance passively diffuse and, almost by accident, bump into the mutated PBP to be able to bind.

This translates to the MIC also becoming higher and higher in SP whose PBPs have more and more mutations. This is due to the fact that, with increasing mutations, there need to be more amoxicillin molecules in the patient so that the accidental amoxicillin-PBP collisions can occur. Therefore, higher amoxicillin doses are needed to overcome this form of resistance. Higher doses (80 to 100 mg/kg/d) are effective, whereas lower doses (40 to 50 mg/kg/d) are not. Further escalation of the dose to much above 100 mg/kg/d is not more effective because the absorption capacity of the gut is saturated above this dose.

Oral Cephalosporins of Little Use

This relative resistance unfortunately is not relevant to oral cephalosporins because the concentrations of these drugs that reached the middle ear, even with the highest doses available, are not high enough to treat organisms with MICs higher than 0.45 mg/L. Unfortunately, at least 90% of MDR pneumococcus have cephalosporin MICs that are higher than this.[2] This makes oral cephalosporins nearly useless in treating MDR pneumococcus.

Table 22-1

Expected Clinical Success (%) Treating MDR 19A
Streptococcus pneumoniae With Acute Otitis Media Antibiotics

HD Amox-icillin	Azithro-mycin	TMP/Sulfa	Clinda-mycin	Oral Cephalo-sporin	Ceftria-xone	Levo-floxacin	Line-zolid
65 to 80	30	<10	60	<10	80	>95	>95

Ceftriaxone

On the other hand, three 50 mg/kg doses of parenteral ceftriaxone have a high likelihood of success (almost 80%; Table 22-1) despite higher cephalosporin MICs up to 4.0 mg/L. This can be given either on 3 consecutive days or every other day over 5 days. This success is due to the fact that serum and middle ear concentrations of ceftriaxone are generally 10 to 20 times higher than those that can be achieved by any oral cephalosporins in any dose.

Clindamycin

MDR pneumococcal strains are susceptible to clindamycin in 50% to 60% of strains using a dose of 10 mg/kg 3 times daily. This drug has an unpleasant taste, to put it mildly, and often must be camouflaged with extra flavorings or mixed in with pudding or chocolate syrup to facilitate administration.

Off-Label Antibiotics for Acute Otitis Media

Both linezolid and levofloxacin have excellent activity against MDR pneumococcus and one would expect more than 95% success with either drug. However, neither drug should be used routinely. Linezolid is quite expensive and can cause bone marrow suppression, particularly beginning in the second week of use. Fatal lactic acidosis can also occur with long-term use. Levofloxacin is relatively safe to use, but routine use will induce resistance and this is a drug we need to hold in reserve and use sparingly. It is advisable to warn parents that they may see information on the Internet that indicates that beagle puppies and fetal rabbits suffer hip dysplasia. Similar issues have not occurred in humans. However, tendinitis and Achilles tendon rupture have been reported.

Until we see whether PCV13 will eliminate most MDR pneumococcus, particularly serotype 19A,[3] treatment choices for MDR pneumococcus likely will be driven by the

MIC if available. Do not be discouraged if the MIC to ceftriaxone, amoxicillin, or penicillin is listed as being "resistant" but is also less than 4.0 mg/L. High-dose amoxicillin or 3 doses of ceftriaxone will produce success in ~80% of these cases. However, if the MIC to ceftriaxone or amoxicillin is greater than or equal to 4.0 mg/L, then use of levofloxacin or linezolid may be necessary. Consider consulting with your local infectious disease expert before using these drugs.

In situations where one does not have susceptibilities but has a high suspicion for MDR pneumococcus, use of high-dose amoxicillin will also most likely be effective. Intramuscular ceftriaxone in 3 doses will provide somewhat higher rates of success and clindamycin will provide somewhat lower rates of success.

References

1. Leibovitz E, Greenberg D, Piglansky L, et al. Recurrent acute otitis media occurring within one month from completion of antibiotic therapy: relationship to the original pathogen. *Pediatr Infect Dis J.* 2003;22(3):209-216.
2. Harrison CJ, Woods C, Stout G, Martin B, Selvarangan R. Susceptibilities of *Haemophilus influenzae, Streptococcus pneumoniae,* including serotype 19A, and *Moraxella catarrhalis* paediatric isolates from 2005 to 2007 to commonly used antibiotics. *J Antimicrob Chemother.* 2009;63(3):511-519.
3. Grijalva CG, Pelton SI. A second-generation pneumococcal conjugate vaccine for prevention of pneumococcal diseases in children. *Curr Opin Pediatr.* 2011;23(1):98-104.

SECTION VII

PHARYNGITIS

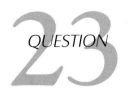

IS A THROAT CULTURE NECESSARY IN THE SETTING OF A NEGATIVE RAPID STREPTOCOCCAL ANTIGEN TEST?

Kevin B. Spicer, MD, PhD, MPH and Preeti Jaggi, MD

Pharyngitis, or sore throat, is a common presenting complaint for acute care visits in pediatrics. Although the majority of cases of acute pharyngitis are associated with viruses, a significant percentage are related to *Streptococcus pyogenes* (Group A streptococcus [GAS]). Data suggest that this percentage can be in the range of 30% to 40% for children who present with acute sore throat.[1] Although strep pharyngitis is a self-limited illness, suppurative (eg, peritonsillar abscess, cervical lymphadenitis) and nonsuppurative complications (eg, acute glomerulonephritis, acute rheumatic fever) can occur. A concern for these complications has led to the emphasis on treatment of acute streptococcal pharyngitis.

Because most cases of pharyngitis are related to viruses and do not require antibiotic therapy, timely and appropriate treatment of GAS pharyngitis necessitates timely and accurate diagnosis. Consequently, one of the most crucial decisions to make in evaluating a patient with pharyngitis is whether to perform a diagnostic test (eg, rapid antigen test and/or bacterial culture). The clinician needs to consider 2 principles: (1) a desire to limit the potential adverse effects to the individual associated with antibiotic treatment, and (2) a desire to limit population exposure to unnecessary antibiotics and thereby decrease the impact of antibiotic overuse as a driving force of antimicrobial resistance.

The best way to limit false-positive errors is to more appropriately test those who present with a complaint of pharyngitis. Clinical and epidemiologic characteristics can be helpful in increasing (or decreasing) the presumed likelihood of streptococcal infection, but history and examination are not sufficient for accurate diagnosis. Pharyngitis that is accompanied by rhinitis, stridor, hoarseness, conjunctivitis, cough, and/or diarrhea is highly likely to have a viral etiology; it is generally unnecessary to perform diagnostic testing for GAS when these symptoms are present. Symptoms such as an abrupt onset of fever, throat pain, headache, abdominal pain, and dysphagia, and signs such as exudative pharyngitis, palatal petechiae, uvulitis, and tender anterior cervical nodes are suggestive

Table 23-1
Sensitivity of Rapid Antigen Detection Tests Relative to Culture

RADT	*Sensitivity, %*	*Specificity, %*
Enzyme immunoassay	80 to 97	93 to 100
Optical immunoassay	75 to 97	89 to 99

Adapted from Bisno AL, Gerber MA, Gwaltney JM, Kaplan EL, Schwartz RH. Practice guidelines for the diagnosis and management of group A streptococcal pharyngitis. *Clin Infect Dis.* 2002;35(3):113-125.

of GAS pharyngitis. In addition, in this context, the absence of rhinitis, hoarseness, conjunctivitis, and cough are more suggestive of GAS pharyngitis. Patients who have symptoms persisting longer than 4 to 5 days at the time of presentation are unlikely to have GAS pharyngitis, as it is a self-limited illness that usually lasts 3 to 5 days.

The traditional criterion standard for diagnosis is the throat culture (ie, culture of throat swab on sheep blood agar plate [BAP]).[2] Proper collection of the throat swab specimen is of utmost importance and requires swabbing of the tonsillar tissue and the posterior pharynx. This can be problematic with the uncooperative child. The primary disadvantage of the throat culture is that it requires 24 to 48 hours and is not particularly useful for making treatment decisions during the office visit. Treatment can be withheld while awaiting culture results without increasing the risk for nonsuppurative complications, as evidence suggests that the risk for acute rheumatic fever is markedly reduced as long as treatment is initiated within 9 days of symptom onset.[3] However, this may delay clinical resolution and allow for ongoing spread of disease. Consequently, rapid antigen detection tests (RADT) have been developed to more quickly identify the organism and allow prompt initiation of therapy. These rapid tests involve detection of the group-specific carbohydrate antigen from the GAS cell wall using a variety of immunologic techniques. RADTs generally have high specificity but variable sensitivity[4] (Table 23-1). Sensitivity and specificity vary depending upon the population of interest, the experience and technical proficiency of the individuals obtaining the throat swabs and performing the tests, and the specifics of the gold standard throat culture (eg, office based versus laboratory based). Molecular tests for more direct detection of the organism from throat specimens have also been developed and may provide a more sensitive and specific alternative to throat culture when only the presence of GAS is of concern.[5] These tests include the GAS D-Test (GenProbe, Inc, San Diego, CA), which utilizes a chemiluminescent DNA probe to detect GAS-specific rRNA sequences, and the LightCycler Strep-A assay (Roche Applied Science, Indianapolis, IN), which utilizes a real-time polymerase chain reaction (PCR) method to detect GAS-specific genetic material. These tests can provide more rapid results than culture but are not office-based assays.

Current recommendations for pediatric patients indicate that negative results on a rapid antigen test for GAS should be followed up by throat culture.[2,6] Whether this is cost-effective and necessary is at least partially dependent upon the baseline rate of GAS and its complications within the population of interest. An individual or practice should evaluate the performance of their rapid test within their population to determine if this recommendation seems warranted. That is, direct comparison of the office-based RADT with culture following standard office practice (ie, office-based culture, hospital-based culture, reference laboratory–based culture) should be performed to determine the performance characteristics of the test within the typical practice of the particular clinical setting. In our own institution, a DNA probe assay (GASDirect Test) has replaced routine culture as the back-up method of GAS detection. The false-negative rate for rapid antigen testing (OSOM Strep A Test—genzyme Diagnostics, Framingham, MA) is 6% to 7% relative to the DNA probe assay (unpublished data). Because no currently available rapid test is perfect (ie, 100% sensitivity, 100% specificity) and the risk of nonsuppurative complications is higher in pediatric patients than in adults, follow-up testing of point-of-care rapid test negative specimens continues to be recommended.

Serologic testing for GAS-relevant antibodies (eg, streptolysin O, deoxyribonuclease B, hyaluronidase, and streptokinase) is not useful in acute infection because antibodies do not increase until weeks after the infection. Such testing, however, is useful in confirming recent infection, which is important in diagnosing GAS sequelae such as acute rheumatic fever and poststreptococcal glomerulonephritis.

References

1. Shaikh N, Leonard E, Martin JM. Prevalence of streptococcal pharyngitis and streptococcal carriage in children: a meta-analysis. *Pediatrics*. 2010;126(3):e557-e564.
2. Bisno AL, Gerber MA, Gwaltney JM, Kaplan EL, Schwartz RH. Practice guidelines for the diagnosis and management of group A streptococcal pharyngitis. *Clin Infect Dis*. 2002;35(3):113-125.
3. Gerber MA, Baltimore RS, Eaton CB, et al. Prevention of rheumatic fever and diagnosis and treatment of acute streptococcal pharyngitis: a scientific statement from the American Heart Association Rheumatic Fever, Endocarditis, and Kawasaki Disease Committee of the Council on Cardiovascular Disease in the Young, the Interdisciplinary Council on Functional Genomics and Translational Biology, and the Interdisciplinary Council on Quality of Care and Outcomes Research. *Circulation*. 2009;119(11):1541-1551.
4. Gerber MA, Shulman ST. Rapid diagnosis of pharyngitis caused by group A streptococci. *Clin Microbiol Rev*. 2004;17(3):571-580.
5. Chapin KC, Blake P, Wilson CD. Performance characteristics and utilization of rapid antigen test, DNA probe, and culture for detection of Group A streptococci in an acute care clinic. *J Clin Microbiol*. 2002;40(11):4207-4210.
6. American Academy of Pediatrics. Group A streptococcal infections. In: Pickering LK, ed. *Red Book: 2009 Report of the Committee on Infectious Diseases*. 28th ed. Elk Grove Village, IL: American Academy of Pediatrics; 2009:616-628. http://aapredbook.aappublications.org/cgi/content/full/2009/1/3.125. Accessed August 12, 2010.

WHAT IS THE BEST TREATMENT OPTION FOR GROUP A STREPTOCOCCAL PHARYNGITIS? WHAT IF THE PATIENT IS ALLERGIC TO BETA-LACTAM ANTIBIOTICS?

Kevin B. Spicer, MD, PhD, MPH and Preeti Jaggi, MD

Group A streptococcal (GAS) pharyngitis is a self-limited illness, with resolution of symptoms typically occurring within 3 to 5 days, even without specific therapy. Therefore, treatment of GAS pharyngitis is directed at prevention of suppurative (eg, peritonsillar abscess, cervical lymphadenitis) and nonsuppurative (eg, acute glomerulonephritis, acute rheumatic fever) complications. Concern for these complications has led to the continued emphasis on treatment of acute GAS pharyngitis. Although there is evidence that treatment can be delayed pending diagnostic evaluation without increasing the risk for nonsuppurative complications, such a delay may prolong the time to clinical resolution and will allow for potential ongoing transmission of infection and spread of disease. However, one also has to weigh the potential impact of treatment in the absence of documented streptococcal infection. Particularly, one needs to consider the potential for adverse effects to the individual and the potential population impact resulting from antimicrobial overuse and increasing resistance.

Once a diagnosis of GAS pharyngitis has been made, antibacterial therapy should be initiated. Because there has been no convincing evidence of in vitro resistance of GAS to penicillin, the drug of choice for GAS pharyngitis remains penicillin.[1,2] However, for ease of administration and palatability, amoxicillin is generally used for those patients who require liquid medication. Recommended duration of therapy with penicillin (PCN)/ amoxicillin remains 10 days and dosing is generally twice a day. A Cochrane review published in 2009 evaluated 20 studies, including more than 13,000 patients with GAS, comparing standard duration (ie, 10 days) of oral penicillin with short duration (ie, 2 to 6 days) of a comparator oral antibiotic.[3] The short duration treatment group had a lower risk of early clinical treatment failure and a lower rate of noncompliance but had a higher rate of medication adverse effects. There was no difference in clinical recurrence, early bacteriologic treatment failure, or late bacteriologic treatment failure (when studies involving low-dose azithromycin were excluded). The authors concluded that shorter courses of therapy have comparable efficacy to the standard 10-day course of penicillin. However, these shorter courses generally involved newer, more expensive, and more broadly active oral antibiotics, which are not currently recommended as first-line agents. Data on the use of shorter courses of therapy with PCN/amoxicillin are not sufficient to recommend a shorter course of therapy with these agents at this time.

Although somewhat controversial, the 2009 Red Book states that single daily dosing of amoxicillin is "an acceptable option if strict adherence to once-daily dosing can be ensured."[1] This is based upon several prospective studies showing equivalent microbiologic eradication after treatment with once-daily amoxicillin versus traditionally dosed penicillin or amoxicillin.[4,5] For example, Clegg et al compared the use of once-daily to twice-daily amoxicillin for treatment of GAS pharyngitis in ~650 children ages 3 to 18.[4] All patients achieved clinical cure and the once-daily group was found noninferior to the twice-daily group in bacteriologic persistence, bacteriologic relapse, and clinical recurrence. Benzathine penicillin G is an alternative if the patient cannot tolerate oral medication or if compliance is of concern.

For the penicillin-allergic patient, a macrolide (eg, erythromycin or azithromycin) is recommended, although up to 10% of GAS may be resistant and rates may be significantly higher in specific geographic areas at given times.[6] If erythromycin is chosen for therapy, the medication should be given for 10 days. However, only 5 days of therapy are needed for azithromycin. Clindamycin is an additional alternative and less than 1% of GAS have historically been resistant in the United States,[7] although much higher rates of resistance have been found in other countries.[8,9] Therefore, it is important to know your local antibiogram data prior to prescribing a macrolide or lincosamide (clindamycin) agent for the treatment of GAS. Additionally, as much higher rates of resistance have been found in other countries, consideration of potential resistance is important when making treatment decisions for the patient who has recently traveled internationally and has signs, symptoms, and testing indicative of GAS.

For the questionable penicillin-allergic patient, or the patient without history of significant urticaria or anaphylaxis, a cephalosporin would be an option, particularly if the patient has been treated for other infections (eg, otitis media) with cephalosporins without incident. A first-generation cephalosporin (with a narrower spectrum of activity) such as cephalexin would be preferable over later generation agents.

References

1. American Academy of Pediatrics. Group A streptococcal infections. In: Pickering LK, ed. *Red Book: 2009 Report of the Committee on Infectious Diseases.* 28th ed. Elk Grove Village, IL: American Academy of Pediatrics; 2009:616–628. http://aapredbook.aappublications.org/cgi/content/full/2009/1/3.125. Accessed August 12, 2010.
2. Gerber MA, Baltimore RS, Eaton CB, et al. Prevention of rheumatic fever and diagnosis and treatment of acute streptococcal pharyngitis: a scientific statement from the American Heart Association Rheumatic Fever, Endocarditis, and Kawasaki Disease Committee of the Council on Cardiovascular Disease in the Young, the Interdisciplinary Council on Functional Genomics and Translational Biology, and the Interdisciplinary Council on Quality of Care and Outcomes Research. *Circulation.* 2009;119:1541-1551.
3. Altamimi S, Khalil A, Khalaiwi KA, Milner RA, Pusic MV, Al Othman MA. Short versus standard duration antibiotic therapy for acute streptococcal pharyngitis in children. *Cochrane Database Syst Rev.* 2009;(1):CD004872.

4. Clegg HW, Ryan AG, Dallas SD, et al. Treatment of streptococcal pharyngitis with once-daily compared with twice-daily amoxicillin. *Pediatr Infect Dis J*. 2006;25(9):761-767.
5. Lennon DR, Farrell E, Martin DR, Stewart JM. Once-daily amoxicillin versus twice-daily penicillin V in group A β-haemolytic streptoccal pharyngitis. *Archives of Disease in Childhood*. 2008;93(6):474-478.
6. Martin JM, Green M, Barbadora KA, Wald ER. Erythromycin-resistant group A streptococci in schoolchildren in Pittsburgh. *N Engl J Med*. 2002;346(16):1200-1206.
7. Richter SS, Heilmann KP, Beekman SE, et al. Macrolide-resistant *Streptococcus pyogenes* in the United States, 2002-2003. *Clin Infect Dis*. 2005;41(5):599-608.
8. Feng L, Lin H, Ma Y, et al. Macrolide-resistant *Streptococcus pyogenes* from Chinese pediatric patients in association with Tn916 transposons family over a 16-year period. *Diagn Microbiol Infect Dis*. 2010;67(4):369-375.
9. Zavadska D, Berzina D, Drukalska L, Pugacova N, Miklasevics E, Gardovska D. Macrolide resistance in group A beta hemolytic Streptococcus isolated from outpatient children in Latvia. *APMIS*. 2010;118(5):366-370.

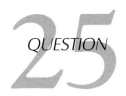

WHY DO WE TREAT STREPTOCOCCAL PHARYNGITIS WHEN IT IS A SELF-LIMITED ILLNESS?

Kevin B. Spicer, MD, PhD, MPH; Preeti Jaggi, MD; and
Angela L. Myers, MD, MPH, FAAP

Group A streptococcal (GAS) pharyngitis is generally a self-limited illness, typically resolving within 3 to 5 days, even without specific treatment. However, suppurative and nonsuppurative complications can occur. Although data on the frequency or likelihood of suppurative complications are limited, it is recognized that such complications are significantly less common now than in the preantibiotic era. Antimicrobial treatment is also beneficial in reducing the duration of symptoms and in decreasing the likelihood of ongoing transmission of infection.

The primary reason to treat GAS pharyngitis is to prevent acute rheumatic fever (ARF). The likelihood of ARF following GAS pharyngitis is quite low and substantially less than the 0% to 3% noted historically in association with epidemics.[1] Various factors have likely been important in this decline in ARF, including improved living conditions in developed countries, the development and widespread use of antibiotics, and a change in circulating strains of GAS (from rheumatogenic to nonrheumatogenic strains). Nevertheless, several localized outbreaks have been reported and sporadic cases continue to occur in the United States and in other developed countries.[2,3] The burden of GAS and ARF (and rheumatic heart disease [RHD]) is substantially higher in the developing world. For example, in sub-Saharan Africa, the prevalence of RHD is reported to be more than 500 per 100,000 children ages 5 to 14 years, whereas in developed countries, the prevalence is less than 50 cases per 100,000 children.[4]

ARF occurs only in the setting of antecedent pharyngeal infection, and typically has a latent period that is in the range of 2 to 4 weeks. Supporting evidence of recent streptococcal infection is required for the diagnosis of ARF (eg, positive rapid antigen test or culture, elevated antibody titer), along with either 2 major or 1 major and 2 minor criteria.[1] An exception to this is the patient who presents with Sydenham chorea, as this clinical

---

Table 25-1

Jones Criteria for Acute Rheumatic Fever

Recent Infection With Group A Streptococcus

- Positive rapid antigen test for GAS
- Positive throat culture for GAS
- Elevated or rising anti-streptolysin O antibody titer
- Elevated or rising anti-DNAse B antibody titer

Major Criteria

- Carditis
- Polyarthritis
- Erythema marginatum
- Subcutaneous nodules
- Chorea

Minor Criteria

- Arthralgia
- Fever
- Elevated acute-phase reactants (eg, C-reactive protein)
- Prolonged PR interval

---

finding alone is diagnostic of rheumatic fever. In this situation, antibody titers are often negative, as the chorea generally occurs weeks to months after the typical latent period when the titers have decreased back to normal/negative values. The major clinical criteria for diagnosis of ARF have been termed the *Jones criteria* and are specifically represented as J = joints, O = heart, N = nodules, E = erythema marginatum, and S = Sydenham chorea, which are listed in Table 25-1. The joint symptoms are noted in ~75% of patients and are migrating in nature, manifesting as pain, swelling, and erythema along with systemic symptoms such as fever, malaise, and anorexia. The hallmark of this feature is resolution in one joint followed by prompt involvement in another. Generally the large joints are involved, with the knee being the most common. Response to nonsteroidal anti-inflammatories is generally dramatic. Carditis occurs in 50% to 60% of cases of ARF and can have a variety of clinical manifestations, from tachycardia and new-onset murmur to fulminant heart failure. Valvulitis, as evidenced by cardiac murmur, is a consistent finding in ARF carditis, whereas myocarditis and pericarditis are more variable. The revised Jones criteria require auscultation of a new valvular murmur in order to meet the criterion of "carditis." Consequently, at this time, echocardiographic finding of valvular regurgitation without a murmur is not sufficient for formal diagnosis. Subcutaneous nodules are seen in patients with severe carditis, but in general are relatively rare, occurring in less than 5% of patients. Lesions are painless and occur over superficial tendons and bony prominences. Erythema marginatum is seen in less than 10% of patients and is distinctive with pink

---

Table 25-2

Proposed Criteria for Diagnosis of Poststreptococcal Reactive Arthritis

A. Characteristics of arthritis
- Acute onset, symmetric or asymmetric, usually nonmigratory, any joint
- Persistent or recurrent symptoms
- No dramatic response to nonsteroidal anti-inflammatory medications

B. Evidence of antecedent GAS infection
C. Does not fulfill modified Jones criteria for ARF

---

macules that coalesce to form a serpiginous pattern. The rash is not painful or pruritic and is usually located on the trunk or extremities.

Additional nonsuppurative complications of streptococcal pharyngitis include poststreptococcal reactive arthritis (PSRA) and poststreptococcal glomerulonephritis (PSGN). These complications are also seen after GAS infection and an intervening latent period. PSRA refers to the clinical situation where arthritis is seen following streptococcal infection, but other criteria for ARF are lacking. The arthritis of PSRA typically occurs 1 to 2 weeks after streptococcal pharyngitis, in contrast to the longer latent period (2 to 4 weeks) associated with ARF. Also, PSRA does not respond as readily to nonsteroidal anti-inflammatory agents as the arthritis associated with ARF. Additionally, the arthritis of PSRA is more likely to be persistent and associated with small joints and the axial skeleton as opposed to the arthritis of ARF, which is more likely to be migratory, transient, and associated with large joints. Although these characteristics may help to differentiate ARF from PSRA, some experts recommend a period of secondary prophylaxis for patients with presumed PSRA and ongoing monitoring for the development of carditis and valvular heart disease. Proposed criteria for the diagnosis of PSRA are provided in Table 25-2.[5]

PSGN generally occurs about 10 days after streptococcal pharyngitis (3 to 4 weeks after streptococcal skin infection). Signs and symptoms include edema, oliguria, hematuria, and hypertension. Edema is typically first noted in the eyelids and progresses variably. Hematuria is present in one-third to half of children with PSGN and has a cola-colored appearance. Hypertension is present in the majority of children, up to 90%, but the severity is variable. Hypertensive encephalopathy, with nausea, vomiting, headaches, and change in mental status, occurs rarely. Although most children present with signs and symptoms of volume overload, including dyspnea, rales, and orthopnea, this is generally a self-limited illness with spontaneous diuresis soon after symptom development. Although there is no evidence that PSGN can be prevented once infection with a nephritogenic strain of GAS has occurred, treatment can prevent transmission of the strain to others and their subsequent development of this complication.

Direct suppurative complications of streptococcal pharyngitis include cervical lymphadenitis, peritonsillar cellulitis, peritonsillar and parapharyngeal abscess, retropharyngeal

---

Table 25-3
Criteria for Streptococcal Toxic Shock Syndrome

Hypotension or shock plus at least 2 of the following:

- Scarlatiniform rash
- Acute respiratory distress syndrome
- Renal impairment
- Hepatic abnormalities
- Disseminated intravascular coagulation
- Soft tissue necrosis

A **definite** case has the above plus isolation of GAS from a **sterile** body site.
A **probable** case has the above plus isolation of GAS from a **nonsterile** body site.

---

abscess, and pneumonia, potentially with empyema.[6,7] These complications should be considered whenever clinical symptoms persist beyond the typical 3 to 5 days. Peritonsillar and parapharyngeal abscesses are more commonly seen in adolescents and are often associated with significant sore throat, dysphagia, trismus, and difficulty in handling normal oral secretions. Retropharyngeal abscesses, in contrast, are more commonly seen in younger children. Clinical presentation is similar to streptococcal pharyngitis, with accompanying hesitancy in moving the neck or readily observable neck hyperextension. Surgical drainage is key to the management of these complications.

Systemic or invasive infection can also occur in the context of streptococcal pharyngitis, which may include bacteremia, osteomyelitis, and endocarditis.[6] Pneumonia associated with GAS can be indistinguishable from community-acquired pneumonias associated with *Streptococcus pneumoniae* and *Staphylococcus aureus* and can also be associated with empyema and necrosis of lung tissue.

Any of the above complications can be associated with toxin-producing strains of GAS, generally *Streptococcus pyogenes* exotoxin A (SPEA), which may lead to streptococcal toxic shock syndrome (STSS). STSS is an acute, severe illness characterized by fever, erythroderma, hypotension, and rapidly developing multiorgan dysfunction/failure (Table 25-3). Evidence of local soft tissue infection with severe pain with rapid progression of infection is common. The hallmark is pain on examination that is out of proportion to visual findings on clinical examination. STSS also occurs without identifiable source of infection, and consequently should be considered in any patient with rapid clinical deterioration and an erythroderma-appearing rash.

Although none of these complications or sequelae of GAS infection are common when considered individually, significant morbidity can be seen when looking at these collectively. Therefore, treatment of GAS infection remains a recommended standard of care as it is nearly impossible to reliably determine, either by clinical or by laboratory findings, an individual's risk of developing a serious or life-threatening complication.

References

1. Gerber MA, Baltimore RS, Eaton CB, et al. Prevention of rheumatic fever and diagnosis and treatment of acute streptococcal pharyngitis: a scientific statement from the American Heart Association Rheumatic Fever, Endocarditis, and Kawasaki Disease Committee of the Council on Cardiovascular Disease in the Young, the Interdisciplinary Council on Functional Genomics and Translational Biology, and the Interdisciplinary Council on Quality of Care and Outcomes Research. *Circulation.* 2009;119(11):1541-1551.
2. Leads from the MMWR: acute rheumatic fever at a Navy training center—San Diego, California. *JAMA.* 1998;259(12):1782-1789.
3. Veasy LG, Wiedmeier SE, Orsmond GS, et al. Resurgence of acute rheumatic fever in the intermountain area of the United States. *N Engl J Med.* 1987;316(8):421-427.
4. Carapetis JR, Steer AC, Mulholland EK, Weber M. The global burden of group A streptococcal diseases. *Lancet Infect Dis.* 2005;5(11):685-694.
5. Ayoub EM, Ahmed S. Update on complications of group A streptococcal infections. *Curr Probl Pediatr.* 1997;27(3):90-101.
6. American Academy of Pediatrics. Group A streptococcal infections. In: Pickering LK, ed. *Red Book: 2009 Report of the Committee on Infectious Diseases.* 28th ed. Elk Grove Village, IL: American Academy of Pediatrics; 2009:616-628. http://aapredbook.aappublications.org/cgi/content/full/2009/1/3.125. Accessed August 12, 2010.
7. Jaggi P, Shulman ST. Group A streptococcal infections. *Pediatr Rev.* 2006;27(3):99-105.

Should I Treat the Asymptomatic Siblings of the Patient Who Has a Positive Rapid Streptococcal Antigen Test?

Kevin B. Spicer, MD, PhD, MPH; Preeti Jaggi, MD; and
Angela L. Myers, MD, MPH, FAAP

In general, when deciding to use antimicrobial therapy, the clinician should consider 2 principles:

1. A desire to limit the potential adverse effects to the individual that may be associated with use of the antimicrobial.
2. A desire to limit the potential adverse effects to the larger population that may result from increasing antimicrobial resistance related to exposure to unnecessary antibiotics.

These principles are considered in the context of a desire to limit the duration and severity of acute illness, to decrease the likelihood of complications of infection, and to reduce ongoing transmission and spread of disease.

With these principles and goals in mind, the clinician's focus should be on maximizing the number of cases of group A streptococcal (GAS) pharyngitis identified and appropriately treated while also minimizing the number of individuals tested and treated who do not have infection. These principles are especially true when considering asymptomatic siblings or other asymptomatic household contacts. Kikuta et al evaluated the role of chemoprophylaxis for siblings of patients with GAS pharyngitis.[1] Siblings receiving antibiotic prophylaxis with either penicillin or a cephalosporin for 3 to 5 days were compared with those receiving no prophylaxis. Within the subsequent 30 days, GAS pharyngitis was diagnosed in 3.0% of the prophylaxis group and in 5.3% of the control (nonprophylaxis) group, a difference that was statistically significant. However, the positive impact of prophylaxis was seen only with cephalosporins (not penicillin) and only if the prophylaxis was continued for 5 days. These authors did not recommend routine prophylaxis given the low rate of infection in sibling contacts, the generally benign course of GAS pharyngitis, and the cost of prophylaxis, both monetarily and in terms of potential adverse drug events and the selection of resistant flora.

Consequently, asymptomatic individuals should generally not be tested or treated, including siblings of those who test positive for GAS.[2,3] It is well known that a significant percentage (10% to 20%) of asymptomatic school-aged children are colonized with GAS, with this number likely toward the upper end of the range when GAS is widespread in the community.[4] Additionally, it is well known that ~25% of household contacts of a patient with GAS pharyngitis will become colonized after exposure. However, only a portion of these individuals will develop disease, with the ultimate risk of disease in contacts being in the range of 5% to 10%. Therefore, testing will fairly often result in positive findings, but this will most often reflect colonization rather than disease. Testing and treating positive findings will then result in a significant amount of inappropriate treatment, or at the very least, these findings will require an extensive and sometimes difficult explanation of carrier status to patients and parents.

Although contacts are at increased risk for infection,[5] asymptomatic siblings should not be routinely tested or treated unless they are at increased risk for disease complications or unless the positive contact has a known nephritogenic or rheumatogenic strain of the organism.[2,3] In this situation, contacts should be tested and then treated if found to be positive. Asymptomatic siblings might also be legitimately tested if the index case has recurrent disease and there is concern that household contacts are involved in the recurrences. In this situation, simultaneous testing and treatment of all positive individuals may have a role in limiting ongoing illness.

Invasive GAS disease is much less common than GAS pharyngitis, occurring in ~3.5/100,000 people in the United States.[6] However, the seriousness of an invasive infection leads to questions regarding the role of prophylaxis for household contacts in this situation. In a study coordinated by the Centers for Disease Control and Prevention (CDC), Robinson et al found an attack rate of 66.1/100,000 for confirmed GAS invasive disease among household contacts of index patients with invasive GAS disease.[6] Although this study did reveal an apparent increased rate of invasive disease (within 1 month of exposure) in household contacts when compared to the general population, the overall risk of invasive disease remained quite low. The attack rate of 66.1/100,000 was based upon one confirmed case of invasive disease occurring among 1514 household contacts. Even in the context of invasive GAS disease, a working group composed of GAS experts has recommended that no routine prophylaxis be administered to household contacts.[7] This recommendation was made because of the low overall risk of invasive disease, the inability to determine those who may be at increased risk, and the lack of a proven prophylactic treatment regimen.

Finally, some families are concerned with the need for testing at the end of a therapeutic course in order to verify bacterial eradication. Such confirmatory testing is not recommended. Follow-up testing would be indicated for individuals with signs and symptoms compatible with refractory streptococcal pharyngitis without clinical features consistent with viral illness. Additionally, follow-up testing would be appropriate for individuals at increased risk for acute rheumatic fever or other complications,[8] which would include those with history of rheumatic fever, those with history of poststreptococcal glomerulonephritis, family members of those with history of these GAS sequelae, individuals with recent varicella infection, and those who are immunosuppressed.

Conclusion

Although some families may push for therapy for asymptomatic family members when one child is diagnosed with GAS pharyngitis, it is helpful for both the clinician and the family to know that there are very few circumstances in which this approach is indicated and that providing therapy to an asymptomatic child, when not indicated, may do more harm than good.

References

1. Kikuta H, Shibata M, Nakata S, et al. Efficacy of antibiotic prophylaxis for intrafamilial transmission of group A b-hemolytic streptococci. *Pediatr Infect Dis J*. 2007;26(2):139-141.
2. American Academy of Pediatrics. Group A streptococcal infections. In: Pickering LK, ed. *Red Book: 2009 Report of the Committee on Infectious Diseases*. 28th ed. Elk Grove Village, IL: American Academy of Pediatrics; 2009:616-628. http://aapredbook.aappublications.org/cgi/content/full/2009/1/3.125. Accessed August 12, 2010.
3. Bisno AL, Gerber MA, Gwaltney JM, Kaplan EL, Schwartz RH. Practice guidelines for the diagnosis and management of group A streptococcal pharyngitis. *Clin Infect Dis*. 2002;35(2):113-125.
4. Shaikh N, Leonard E, Martin JM. Prevalence of streptococcal pharyngitis and streptococcal carriage in children: a meta-analysis. *Pediatrics*. 2010;126(3):e557-e564.
5. Pichichero ME. Treatment and prevention of streptococcal tonsillopharyngitis. In: Basow DS, ed. *UpToDate. 2012*. Waltham, MA: UpToDate.
6. Robinson KA, Rothrock G, Phan Q, et al. Risk for severe group A streptococcal disease among patients' household contacts. *Emerg Infect Dis*. 2003;9(4):443-447.
7. The Prevention of Invasive Group A Streptococcal Infections Workshop Participants. Prevention of invasive group A streptococcal disease among household contacts of case patients and among postpartum and post-surgical patients: recommendations from the Centers for Disease Control and Prevention. *Clin Infect Dis*. 2002; 35(8):950-959.
8. Gerber MA, Baltimore RS, Eaton CB, et al. Prevention of rheumatic fever and diagnosis and treatment of acute streptococcal pharyngitis: a scientific statement from the American Heart Association Rheumatic Fever, Endocarditis, and Kawasaki Disease Committee of the Council on Cardiovascular Disease in the Young, the Interdisciplinary Council on Functional Genomics and Translational Biology, and the Interdisciplinary Council on Quality of Care and Outcomes Research. *Circulation*. 2009;119(11):1541-1551.

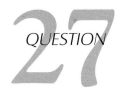
WHAT ARE THE BEST CLINICAL INDICATORS THAT MY PATIENT MAY HAVE STREPTOCOCCAL PHARYNGITIS?

Kevin B. Spicer, MD, PhD, MPH and Preeti Jaggi, MD

Pharyngitis, or sore throat, is a common presenting complaint for acute care visits in pediatrics. Although the majority of cases of acute pharyngitis are nonstreptococcal in etiology, 30% to 40% of children who present with acute sore throat will have *Streptococcus pyogenes* (Group A streptococcus [GAS]) as the etiologic agent.[1] Although streptococcal pharyngitis is a self-limited illness, suppurative and nonsuppurative complications can occur, which has resulted in an emphasis upon accurate and timely diagnosis and treatment of those individuals diagnosed with acute streptococcal disease.

In order to more appropriately manage our patients who present with pharyngitis, we need to optimally evaluate and test so that we can treat in a manner that will maximize outcomes and limit potential complications. Complications can result both from lack of appropriate antimicrobial treatment of streptococcal disease (eg, peritonsillar abscess, acute rheumatic fever) and from inappropriate antimicrobial treatment of nonstreptococcal disease (eg, drug reactions or other drug-associated adverse events). Additionally, inappropriate treatment of viral infections with antimicrobial agents has in large part contributed to the rise of antibiotic resistance nationally, as well as globally. It is important to make the assessment process as time and cost efficient as possible, which necessitates optimizing the use of diagnostic strategies and testing.

The relatively poor clinical accuracy of physicians in diagnosing streptococcal pharyngitis is well recognized.[2,3] Errors include both false-negative diagnoses (ie, diagnosing nonstreptococcal disease when GAS disease is present) and more commonly, false-positive diagnoses (ie, diagnosing GAS disease when nonstreptococcal disease is present). Both can be problematic, with the former increasing the risk of complications to the patient and the latter resulting in unnecessary antibiotic use. The difficulty of accurately estimating likelihood of GAS pharyngitis was illustrated in a study by Poses et al.[3] Physicians who based their diagnosis on clinical examination findings alone overestimated the likelihood of GAS disease in more than 80% of the patients tested. Although no individual sign or symptom is sufficient to make a highly accurate diagnosis, a combination of such signs and symptoms can significantly increase the likelihood of streptococcal disease and allow us to more appropriately target our diagnostic testing (eg, rapid antigen detection test, throat culture). A number of investigators have attempted to determine which clinical sign and symptom combinations are most indicative of infection with GAS.[2,4-7] Historically important in this regard is the *Centor score*, which resulted from a study published in 1981 that evaluated the diagnostic probability of GAS pharyngitis in patients with a combination of 4 clinical features: tonsillar exudates, swollen tender anterior cervical nodes, history of fever, and lack of cough. Patients with all 4 features were found to have a 56% probability of a positive throat culture, whereas the probability of a positive culture ranged from 2.5% to 32% in those with 0 to 3 features. The results of this study have led to the use of the Centor score as an aid to medical decision making in terms of performing diagnostic testing in adult patients. The original scoring system has been modified for pediatrics with the inclusion of age (+1 for age 3 to 14) as another feature to be used in determining the score. McIsaac et al, in a study published in 2004, evaluated patients with at least 2 clinical features of GAS, who were considered to have high enough pretest likelihood of GAS to warrant diagnostic testing.[8] Nearly 70% of children with a modified Centor score of 4 or 5 had a throat culture positive for GAS, indicating that this tool provided better predictive value in children than in adults. Unfortunately, this study did not evaluate the utility of using the scoring system in conjunction with rapid antigen testing followed by culture for those with negative results, which is the current standard of care for the diagnosis of GAS pharyngitis in children. However, the strength of the Centor score and its subsequent modifications, as well as other scoring systems, has been to help determine those patients who should not be tested rather than to make the diagnosis of GAS pharyngitis, as these scoring systems have low specificity. Consequently, we can avoid testing those with low likelihood of disease (in an attempt to limit inappropriate antibiotic use and potential adverse events) and increase our pretest probability of disease and the predictive power of the testing that we do perform. Attempts to develop clinical scoring systems have continued to highlight the significant overlap of clinical signs and symptoms among patients with streptococcal versus nonstreptococcal disease.

Scoring systems that rely on features from history and examination continue to play an important role in improving clinical diagnostic accuracy.[5-7] Although current specifics of these schemes vary, most recognize the following features as important: age (eg, greater than 5 years as opposed to younger than 5 years), abnormal pharynx (which can include marked erythema and/or exudates), abnormal anterior cervical nodes, and, notably, absence of typical features of viral illness (eg, cough, rhinorrhea, hoarseness, diarrhea; Table 27-1). Additional important features to consider include close contact with an individual with documented streptococcal infection, season of the year, acute onset of symptoms, history of significant fever, complaint of sore throat and/or possibly headache, presence of scarlatiniform rash, and palatal petechiae. Streptococcal disease is found to be significantly less likely in the presence of indicators of possible viral illness, such as cough, rhinorrhea, conjunctivitis, hoarseness, and diarrhea.

Scoring systems have also been shown to be useful in limiting inappropriate antibiotic use in resource limited settings. A recent scoring system was developed based upon age,

Table 27-1

Features Associated With Streptococcal Disease

- Marked pharyngeal erythema
- Pharyngeal exudates
- Enlarged, tender anterior cervical nodes
- Palatal petechiae
- Scarlatiniform rash
- Acute onset of symptoms
- Absence of
  - Cough
  - Rhinorrhea
  - Conjunctivitis
  - Hoarseness
  - Diarrhea
- Age greater than 5 years
- Season of the year (occurrence in winter and spring)

"bacterial" signs (ie, tender cervical node, headache, petechia on the palate, abdominal pain, sudden onset) and "viral" signs (ie, conjunctivitis, coryza, diarrhea).[7] This scoring system was also reasonably successful in identifying those most likely to have streptococcal disease and to need antibiotic therapy. Again, these history and clinical features did not allow sufficiently accurate diagnosis so that treatment was fully optimized, especially if considered for use in an environment with more readily available specific diagnostic testing. However, as previously stated, this kind of approach may allow us to better target our diagnostic procedures and make more appropriate use of our time and resources.

References

1. Shaikh N, Leonard E, Martin JM. Prevalence of streptococcal pharyngitis and streptococcal carriage in children: a meta-analysis. *Pediatrics.* 2010;126(3):e557-e564.
2. Centor RM, Witherspoon JM, Dalton HP, Brody CE, Link K. The diagnosis of strep throat in adults in the emergency room. *Med Decis Making.* 1981;1(3):239-246.
3. Poses RM, Cebul RD, Collins M, Fager SS. The accuracy of experienced physicians' probability estimates for patients with sore throat: implications for decision making. *JAMA.* 1985;254(7):925-929.
4. Stillerman M, Bernstein SH. Streptococcal pharyngitis: evaluation of clinical syndromes in diagnosis. *Am J Dis Child.* 1961;101(4):96-109.
5. Breese BB. A simple scorecard for the tentative diagnosis of streptococcal pharyngitis. *Am J Dis Child.* 1977;131(5):514-517.
6. Wald ER, Green MD, Schwartz B, Barbadora K. A streptococcal score card revisited. *Pediatr Emerg Care.* 1998;14(2):109-111.
7. Joachim L, Campos D, Smeesters PR. Pragmatic scoring system for pharyngitis in low-resource settings. *Pediatrics.* 2010;126(3):e1-e7.
8. McIsaac WJ, Kellner JD, Aufricht P, Vanjaka A, Low DE. Empirical validation of guidelines for the management of pharyngitis in children and adults. *JAMA.* 2004;291(13):1587-1595.

SECTION VIII

VIRAL TESTING

How Sensitive and Specific Are the Office-Based Rapid Respiratory Syncytial Virus and Rapid Influenza Tests?

Rebecca C. Brady, MD

Laboratory testing for respiratory syncytial virus (RSV) and/or influenza is recommended when the result will be used to guide patient care. Examples include decisions on initiation of antiviral or antibiotic treatments, impact on other diagnostic testing, and infection control practices. Test results are influenced by the pretest probability that the patient has the viral infection based on his or her signs and symptoms, the epidemiology of infection in the population being tested, and the sensitivity and specificity of the screening test as compared to a criterion standard. Sensitivity is the percentage of the time the test will provide a positive result in the setting of "true infection cases." Specificity is the percentage of the time the test will provide a negative result in the setting of "true no infection cases."

The prevalence of RSV and influenza infections varies. Diagnostic tests are most likely to be truly positive (have a higher sensitivity) during periods of peak viral activity in the population tested. During the off-season, a positive screening test result is most likely to be a false positive and therefore, a confirmatory or criterion standard test should be considered.

For many years, cell (tissue) culture was considered the criterion standard test for diagnosing RSV and influenza infections. More recently, reverse transcriptase-polymerase chain reaction (RT-PCR) has become the new criterion standard test for respiratory virus detection because it has high sensitivity and specificity and results are available in hours as compared to days for cell culture. However, RT-PCR requires laboratory technicians and expensive equipment. In contrast, office-based rapid diagnostic tests offer the advantages of ease of use, cost-effectiveness, and the availability of a result in 10 to 30 minutes. Their sensitivity and/or specificity are usually lower than criterion standard tests, and this should be considered when interpreting results.

Rapid Respiratory Syncytial Virus Tests

RSV is the most common cause of respiratory illness in infants younger than 1 year. Nearly all children have been infected at least once by their second birthday. RSV usually occurs in annual epidemics during the winter and early spring in temperate climates. Spread among household and childcare contacts is common. The period of viral shedding usually is 3 to 8 days. Shedding may last several weeks in young infants or in patients with compromised immune systems.

Laboratory diagnosis of RSV is based on the detection of virus in respiratory secretions. In general, children have higher concentrations of RSV in their secretions (several logs) than adults. Nasal washes or aspirates and nasopharyngeal (NP) or nasal swabs are all acceptable specimens. However, nasal washes or aspirates are usually preferred because they contain more virus than NP or nasal swabs. Specimens should be obtained as close to illness onset as possible, preferably within 5 days after symptom onset. Available rapid antigen-based diagnostic assays include indirect and direct immunofluorescent antibody tests, enzyme-linked immunoassays (EIAs), direct immunoassay, and optical immunoassay. Of these rapid tests, EIAs usually have the best combination of sensitivity, specificity, and ease of use. The sensitivity of EIAs varies from 59% to 97%, although most are in the 80% to 90% range. Specificity varies from 75% to 100%, and both sensitivity and specificity are dependent on the quality of the specimen, the virus and strain being detected, and the manufacturer of the test kit. These tests are most useful for infants with moderate or severe illness. In this setting, they allow for a rapid diagnosis and thereby, additional testing and unnecessary therapies may possibly be avoided.

Rapid Influenza Tests

Influenza is an acute, highly contagious, febrile respiratory illness that occurs in epidemics of varying severity in the winter months. During community outbreaks, schoolchildren have the highest attack rates. Pandemics occur infrequently, but as evidenced in 2009, peak viral activity may be in the warmer months. Viral shedding in nasal secretions usually peaks within the first 3 days of illness and is correlated directly with the degree of fever.

Laboratory diagnosis of influenza is also based on the detection of virus in respiratory secretions. Infants may shed influenza viruses for more than or equal to 1 week. In infants and young children, optimal specimens are nasal aspirates and swabs. In older children and adults, NP aspirates and swabs are preferred specimens. If possible, specimens should be collected during the first 72 hours of illness, as viral shedding decreases rapidly beyond this point.

Rapid influenza diagnostic tests are based on either (1) immunoassay (antibodies bind to the viral nucleoprotein; this reaction is detected by a color change) or (2) viral neuraminidase detection (neuraminidase catalyzes a chemical reaction, which is detected by a color change). Rapid tests differ by the types of respiratory specimens considered acceptable for testing, and therefore the package insert and manufacturer's instructions should be followed. They may or may not distinguish between influenza A and B virus infections. Rapid tests do not identify the subtype of influenza A, and certain subtypes such as the 2009 H1N1 pandemic influenza virus may be harder to detect. Overall, they are

Table 28-1
Rapid Respiratory Syncytial Virus and Influenza Diagnostic Tests

Test	Sensitivity	Specificity
RSV EIA[1,2]	59% to 97% (usually 80% to 90%)	75% to 100%
RSV indirect/direct immunofluorescent antibody tests[1,2]	93% to 98%	92% to 97%
Influenza immunoassay[3,4]	70% to 90% (children) 40% to 60% (adults)	>90%
Influenza neuraminidase detection[3,4]	70% to 90% (children) <40% to 60% (adults)	60% to 90%

approximately 50% to 70% sensitive for detecting influenza and greater than 90% specific. Therefore, false-negative results are more common than false-positive results, especially during peak influenza activity. Follow-up testing with RT-PCR or viral culture should be considered to confirm negative test results. Despite these limitations, rapid tests provide clinicians with prompt results to guide appropriate use of antiviral agents for treatment of influenza in persons with chronic medical conditions who are at increased risk for associated complications.

Office-based rapid RSV and rapid influenza tests (Table 28-1) provide prompt results that contribute to clinical decision making and management. Not all individuals with these suspected viral infections need diagnostic testing. Testing is best reserved for use among high-risk populations during peak viral activity. To properly interpret test results, clinicians should understand their sensitivity and specificity. Rapid tests do not substitute for clinical judgment and experience.

References

1. Henrickson KJ, Hall CB. Diagnostic assays for respiratory syncytial virus diseases. *Pediatr Infect Dis J.* 2007;26(11 suppl):S36-S40.
2. Principi N, Esposito S. Antigen-based assays for the identification of influenza virus and respiratory syncytial virus: why and how to use them in pediatric practice. *Clin Lab Med.* 2009;29(4):649-660.
3. Centers for Disease Control and Prevention. Influenza symptoms and laboratory diagnostic procedures. http://www.cdc.gov/flu/professionals/diagnosis/labprocedures.htm. Accessed September 9, 2010.
4. Harper SA, Bradley JS, Englund JA, et al. Expert Panel of the Infectious Diseases Society of America. Seasonal influenza in adults and children--diagnosis, treatment, chemoprophylaxis, and institutional outbreak management: Clinical practice guidelines of the Infectious Diseases Society of America. *Clin Infect Dis.* 2009;48(8):1003-1032.

Suggested Reading

Ezeanolue E, Ezeanolue C, Dashefsky B. Rapid diagnostic tests for infectious diseases suitable for office use. *Pediatr Rev.* 2005;26(10):383-387.

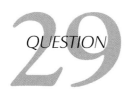

IF I HAVE A 3-MONTH-OLD INFANT IN THE OFFICE WITH RESPIRATORY SYMPTOMS AND NEGATIVE VIRAL TESTING, SHOULD I PROCEED WITH A SEPSIS EVALUATION?

Archana Chatterjee, MD, PhD

The diagnosis of a respiratory viral infection cannot necessarily be ruled out based on laboratory evaluation, particularly with rapid testing. Traditionally, the isolation of respiratory viruses in tissue culture has been the gold standard for confirmation of an infection. However, these methods are time consuming and results are often not available for several days. For a 3-month-old infant, decisions for further evaluation are often based on more rapid methods in vogue today, including commercial rapid diagnostic tests, direct and indirect immunofluorescence antibody tests, and molecular diagnostic methods such as polymerase chain reaction (PCR). Each of these methods has its own sensitivity, specificity, and positive and negative predictive value. Clinicians need to familiarize themselves with the performance characteristics of the test used in order to interpret the results. In general, in the office setting, sophisticated testing methods such as PCR are not likely to be available.

Commercially available rapid diagnostic tests vary in their reliability but are generally between 70% and 90% sensitive and more than 90% specific. One exception to this has been the H1N1 influenza virus rapid antigen test, which confers a sensitivity of 50%. This is not better than a flip of a coin, and as such, is not a good tool to determine whether or not a patient has this strain of influenza A virus. Additionally, both false-positive and false-negative results may be obtained, depending upon the time of year that the test is performed (whether or not the test is being performed in season), duration of the illness (the ability to identify the virus is inversely proportional to the length of time the patient has been ill), adequacy of the clinical sample (for some viruses it is important to obtain epithelial cells as well as mucus), and the type of virus for which the test is done (some viruses are more easily identified than others).

The decision to proceed with a sepsis evaluation should be made based upon the clinical presentation as well as the probability that the illness is associated with a respiratory viral illness. For example, in a patient who is febrile, irritable, somnolent, or feeding poorly, irrespective of the test results for viral etiologies, the clinician should consider pursuing a sepsis evaluation. In other patients who only have respiratory symptoms, the decision is more difficult. A few published studies suggest that the rates of concomitant serious bacterial infections (SBIs) in young infants with a positive respiratory syncytial virus (RSV) antigen test are low. The exception appears to be urinary tract infections (UTIs), which do sometimes occur in young infants who are RSV positive by rapid testing. The suggestion has therefore been made that while full sepsis evaluations may not be necessary in nontoxic-appearing infants with a positive RSV test result, it may be prudent to evaluate their urine for a clinically relevant UTI.

A number of studies with differing designs and populations of children have addressed the issue of interpreting rapid influenza tests in the context of the risk of concomitant SBIs. A good review of these studies concludes that in the well-appearing, fully vaccinated febrile infant, given the declining rate of occult bacteremia, blood cultures may not be necessary in influenza-positive children. A more recent multicenter, prospective, cross-sectional study during 3 consecutive influenza seasons at 5 pediatric emergency departments confirms the low risk of SBI in influenza-positive infants (2.5%) compared to those who were influenza negative (13.3%). There was also a lower risk of UTIs (2.4%) in influenza-positive infants compared to those who tested negative (10.8%). Thus, it appears that in nontoxic-appearing infants who are influenza positive, a sepsis evaluation may not be necessary, but a urinalysis and culture may be useful.

Another aspect of the question posed that is not directly related to the test results or the patient's clinical status, but has a bearing on the clinician's decision, is his or her familiarity with the patient's family. The physician may choose to observe a patient with respiratory symptoms and negative viral testing, if he/she knows the family well and trusts the judgment of the caregivers. On the other hand, when the same patient is from a family that is new to the practice, or if the clinician is not confident about his or her ability to assess the patient, he or she may elect to pursue the sepsis evaluation.

There are further caveats to the conclusions in the paragraphs above. An association between influenza virus infections and bacterial infections has been recognized for nearly 100 years. It is important to understand, however, that these tend to be secondary and not concomitant infections. Several studies have determined that the rate of SBI coexisting with influenza disease was low. However, the diagnosis of influenza in these studies was often in older children and based on cell culture confirmation. Thus, there appears to be insufficient evidence to change current clinical practice algorithms for young infants with respiratory symptoms, particularly if they are febrile, based on office-based viral testing. Ultimately, the decision to initiate a sepsis evaluation must rest with the skilled clinician, who needs to weigh the clinical data and incorporate his or her knowledge of the performance characteristics of rapid viral testing before determining an appropriate course of action.

Suggested Readings

Krief WI, Levine DA, Platt SL, et al. Influenza virus infection and the risk of serious bacterial infections in young febrile infants. *Pediatrics*. 2009;124(1):30-39.

Levine DA, Platt SL, Dayan PS, et al. Risk of serious bacterial infection in young febrile infants with respiratory syncytial virus infections. *Pediatrics*. 2004;113(6):1728-1734.

Titus MO, Wright SW. Prevalence of serious bacterial infections in febrile infants with respiratory syncytial virus infection. *Pediatrics*. 2003;112(2):282-284.

Vega R. Rapid viral testing in the evaluation of the febrile infant and child. *Curr Opin Pediatr*. 2005;17(3):363-367.

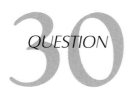
If I Have a 5-Week-Old Infant With Positive Rapid Viral Testing Who Does Not Need Hospital Admission, Is a Sepsis Evaluation Necessary?

Archana Chatterjee, MD, PhD

There are 3 important aspects to this question:

1. Whether the positive rapid viral test can be relied upon to diagnose a true viral infection in very young infants.
2. Whether a very young infant is likely to have a concomitant serious bacterial infection (SBI).
3. How well the clinician who is making the decision about further testing knows the patient and family.

To answer the first question, it is important to define what rapid viral testing means. Currently, rapid viral tests could include commercial rapid antigen-detection tests, direct and indirect immunofluorescence antibody assays, or molecular-based tests such as polymerase chain reaction (PCR). Many offices perform or have ready access to rapid antigen-detection tests, while immunofluorescence testing is offered less often, and more sophisticated testing methods such as PCR are not available in physician offices. However, hospital-based clinics and emergency rooms (ERs) may have access to such rapid testing. Although PCR assays are relatively "rapid," most still require hours to days for results. Each of these tests has its own performance characteristics, including sensitivity, specificity, and positive and negative predictive value. Clinicians using these tests need to be familiar with reliability of the particular test they are ordering in order to interpret the results accurately. Other commercially available rapid diagnostic tests that can be used at the bedside vary in their reliability. Depending upon the time of year that the test is performed, duration of the presenting illness, adequacy of the clinical sample, and the type of virus for which the test is done, both false-positive and false-negative results may be obtained. Thus, the answer to the question posed in the vignette may partly be based upon the location of the clinician (office- versus hospital-based clinic or ER), familiarity with the test characteristics, and other factors as delineated above.

The second question relates to the host's status rather than the accuracy of the viral rapid diagnostic test. As the vignette stipulates that this young infant does not need hospital admission, one can presume that overt signs and symptoms of sepsis such as temperature instability, hypotension, inconsolable irritability, somnolence, or poor feeding are absent. The question that arises then is the probability of a concomitant SBI in this case. There are some articles that report that the rates of concurrent SBIs are low in young infants with a positive rapid respiratory syncytial virus (RSV) antigen test. However, these studies indicate that urinary tract infections (UTIs) can sometimes occur simultaneously in young infants who are RSV positive by rapid antigen testing. Therefore, it has been suggested that in nontoxic-appearing infants with a positive rapid RSV test result, it may be advisable to perform a urinalysis and culture for a clinically relevant UTI. In such cases, a full sepsis evaluation of the infant may not be necessary.

Rapid influenza testing is also commonly obtained in young infants who present with acute illness during influenza season. The results of such tests can be applied to the management of these patients based on the data from a few peer-reviewed articles. In a study done by the Texas Children's Hospital Emergency Department over 4 influenza seasons, the odds of SBI including pneumonia in patients ages 29 to 90 days if they were influenza positive were 79% less than if they were influenza negative. For SBIs excluding pneumonia, the odds in influenza-positive patients were 81% less than in influenza-negative patients. In other words, if a young infant was positive for influenza A, it was highly unlikely that he or she also had an SBI at the same time. A more recently published multicenter, prospective, cross-sectional study conducted at 5 pediatric emergency departments (EDs) during 3 consecutive influenza seasons confirms the low risk of SBI in influenza-positive infants (2.5%) compared to those who were influenza negative (13.3%). In this study, there was a small, but significantly lower risk of UTIs (2.4%) in influenza-positive infants compared to those who tested negative (10.8%). Therefore, in young, nontoxic-appearing infants who are influenza positive, a urinalysis and culture may be useful, but a full sepsis evaluation may not be needed.

The third facet to the question that is not directly related to either the test results or the patient's clinical status, but has an important impact on the clinician's decision regarding further evaluation, is his or her familiarity with the patient's family. If the family is well-known to and trusted by the clinician, he or she may elect to forego a sepsis evaluation in a nontoxic-appearing young infant with positive rapid viral testing. However, if the same patient comes from a family that is new to the practice, or if the clinician does not trust the judgment of the caregivers, the more prudent course may be to complete a sepsis evaluation even with a positive rapid viral test.

Conclusion

Positive rapid viral testing can be a useful aid in further diagnostic decision making for young infants. However, sound clinical judgment should always be used when deciding about the need for a sepsis evaluation in a young infant who is ill. In order to make the best choice for the patient, the clinician needs to be knowledgeable about the validity of the positive rapid viral test in the context of the clinical presentation.

Suggested Readings

Krief WI, Levine DA, Platt SL, et al. Influenza virus infection and the risk of serious bacterial infections in young febrile infants. *Pediatrics*. 2009;124(1):30-39.

Levine DA, Platt SL, Dayan PS, et al. Risk of serious bacterial infection in young febrile infants with respiratory syncytial virus infections. *Pediatrics*. 2004;113(6):1728-1734.

Smitherman HF, Caviness AC, Macias CG. Retrospective review of serious bacterial infections in infants who are 0 to 36 months of age and have Influenza A infection. *Pediatrics*. 2005;115(3);710-718.

Titus MO, Wright SW. Prevalence of serious bacterial infections in febrile infants with respiratory syncytial virus infection. *Pediatrics*. 2003; 112(2):282-284.

SECTION IX

DIARRHEA

WHEN ARE ANTIBIOTICS INDICATED FOR A CHILD WITH A BACTERIAL CAUSE OF DIARRHEA?

Amber Hoffman, MD

There are 2 million deaths annually from acute diarrhea worldwide. The majority are caused by viral infections, for which there is only supportive treatment available. Bacterial diarrhea accounts for 2% to 10% of childhood diarrheal disease in developed countries. Common causes of bacterial diarrhea in the United States are *Shigella spp*, *Salmonella spp*, enterohemorrhagic *Escherichia coli* (EHEC), *Campylobacter spp*, *Yersinia enterocolitica*, and *Clostridium difficile*.[1] Conditions putting patients at higher risk include HIV positivity, sickle cell disease, diabetes, and immunodeficiency or immune suppression.[1] Neonates and young infants, as well as previously healthy hosts with severe cholera, shigellosis, or typhoid fever, are also in this higher risk group. Treatment may also decrease the transmission of disease to secondary contacts and potentially impact the number of cases in an outbreak.[2]

Children who present with suspected bacterial enteritis often have abdominal pain, hematochezia, and fever. The question then arises as to whether to treat before a pathogen is confirmed, or whether to treat them with antibiotics at all. The threats of increasing bacterial resistance should be taken into consideration. Treatment also can cause eradication of normal, protective gastrointestinal (GI) flora, leading to superinfection. Risks of induction of disease from Shiga-toxin–producing bacteria, as well as adverse drug reactions from the antibiotics themselves, are also considerations. The balance of these risks must be weighed against the threat of the bacterial gastroenteritis itself, as well as the control of widespread outbreaks. This balance differs based on the region of the world and even local resistance patterns and epidemiology.[2]

The World Health Organization recommends empiric antimicrobial therapy in the setting of febrile, acute, and bloody diarrhea in young children. However, much of the acute infectious diarrhea is viral in nature, or self-limited, regardless of its etiology. As a result, each case should be evaluated independently, if possible, taking into consideration the patient's unique characteristics, local epidemiology and incidence of bacterial enteritis, as well as local antibiotic resistance patterns. A majority of patients do not require laboratory evaluation for acute diarrhea and can be managed as outpatients. Those with severe illness requiring hospitalization may benefit from laboratory evaluations, stool culture, and supportive care. Negative cultures do not exclude the possibility of bacterial infection. Mixed infections also occur.[2]

The decision to start empiric antibiotics usually takes place based solely on clinical grounds or local outbreaks given the time it takes for stool culture results to return. Some of the clinical features that may help with guiding antibiotic implementation are intense tenesmus with *Shigella*; mimicry of appendicitis with *Yersinia*; painless, copious watery diarrhea associated with *Vibrio cholera*; and severe bloody diarrhea in patients with *E coli*. Diarrhea that begins after antibiotic exposure or exposure to elderly, hospitalized adults, should raise a suspicion for *C difficile*. See Table 31-1 for some of the common sources of bacterial enteritis and severe clinical presentations.[3-10]

If deciding to use antibiotics, one should take into consideration the risk of the antibiotics themselves in pediatric patients. Tetracyclines remain limited in pediatrics due to permanent dental discoloration, enamel hypoplasia, and impaired bone growth side effects. They are rarely, if ever, utilized as a treatment option in children younger than 8 years for diarrheal illness in the United States. Fluoroquinolones are only recommended for use in children younger than 18 years in a limited number of settings, due to concerns of cartilage damage. However, in developing countries, areas of high resistance, or areas with limited resources, the potential benefits of antibiotic therapy may outweigh the side effects of the antibiotics themselves.[2]

Antibiotic treatment is recommended for patients with severe disease or underlying immunosuppression with *Shigella* species infections. Empiric therapy while awaiting culture, or antibiotic use in mild disease, is primarily to prevent spread of disease, as ingestion of 10 to 100 organisms is sufficient to cause disease. Knowledge of local resistance patterns is needed as 80% of *Shigella* may be resistant to ampicillin and 40% to trimethoprim-sulfamethoxazole (TMP-SMX). Cefixime may be given orally to children as outpatients keeping in mind that there are high resistance rates in adults with shigellosis. Azithromycin currently has an advantage of low resistance rates, easy dosing, and a safe adverse event profile in pediatric patients.[4]

In *Salmonella*, antibiotic treatment can prolong the shedding period and is therefore not usually indicated in noninvasive disease. However, children younger than 3 months, those with chronic GI disease, hemoglobinopathy, or other immune-suppressive conditions should be treated. For at-risk patients, ampicillin, amoxicillin, or TMP-SMX could be used for susceptible strains. If resistance patterns are high, ceftriaxone, cefotaxime, azithromycin, or fluoroquinolones could be considered. With localized invasive disease, empiric therapy with ceftriaxone or cefotaxime may be used. For invasive disease, a 10- to 14-day course is recommended. Chronic *Salmonella typhi* carriage is unusual in children but may be eradicated by high-dose parenteral ampicillin, oral amoxicillin with probenecid, or ciprofloxaxin for adults. Chloramphenicol has had increasing resistance rates as well as a risk of side effects. It is still used empirically in typhoid fever in some countries and is associated with decreased mortality.[5]

Campylobacter jejuni and *Campylobacter coli* infections have mild infection lasting 1 to 2 days typically, but prolonged infection with relapses mimicking inflammatory bowel disease can occur. Erythromycin and azithromycin shorten duration of illness and excretion of the organism from stool and can prevent relapse when given early. There

Table 31-1

Bacterial Gastroenteritis Presentations, Complications, and Sources of Infection[4-10]

Bacteria	Common Sources of Infection	Common Presentations	Severe Complications and Less Common Presentations
Campylobacter spp	• Farm animals • Meat sources • Young dogs, cats hamsters, birds • Undercooked poultry • Untreated water • Unpasteurized milk • Poultry carcasses	Diarrhea, abdominal pain, malaise, fever, hematochezia	• Mimics appendicitis, intussusception, inflammatory bowel disease • Acute idiopathic polyneuritis, Miller Fisher syndrome, Reiter syndrome, and erythema nodosum
Escherichia coli	• Ground beef • Unpasteurized milk • Contaminated water or apple cider • Petting zoos • Raw fruits and vegetables	• Hematochezia, abdominal pain, fever • Watery stools with cramping	• Hemolytic uremic syndrome • Thrombotic thrombocytopenic purpura
Salmonella spp	• Poultry, livestock, reptiles, and pets • Contaminated beef, eggs, dairy • Outbreaks from foods contaminated by infected animals or humans have included fruits, vegetables, peanut butter, frozen pot pies, infant formula, cereal, and bakery products • Typhoid—Humans with direct contact to infected individual	• Diarrhea, abdominal pain, abdominal cramps, fever • Typhoid fever— bacteremia, fever, headache, malaise, anorexia, and lethargy, abdominal pain and tenderness, hepatomegaly, splenomegaly, rose spots, change in mental status • Diarrhea common in children	• Bacteremia • Osteomyelitis • Meningitis • Treatment can prolong shedding period • Typhoid— Uncommon in USA— 400 cases per year, endemic in other countries • Treatment can prolong shedding period

(continued)

Table 31-1 (continued)

Bacterial Gastroenteritis Presentations, Complications, and Sources of Infection[4-10]

Bacteria	Common Sources of Infection	Common Presentations	Severe Complications and Less Common Presentations
Shigella spp	• Fecal-oral with person-to-person contact or with contaminated object • Contaminated food or water • Sexual contact	• S sonnei—watery diarrhea • S flexneri, S boydii, and S dysenteria—fever, hematochezia, tenesmus, mucoid stools, and abdominal pain	• Reiter syndrome • Hemolytic—Uremic Syndrome • Toxic megacolon and intestinal perforation • Toxic encephalopathy (Ekiri syndrome)
Yersinia spp	• Principal reservoir is swine • Contaminated pork or tofu • Unpasteurized milk Cross contamination with handling of raw pork • Chitterlings	• Fever and diarrhea • Leukocytes, blood, and mucus in stool	• Bacteremia, pharyngitis, meningitis, osteomyelitis, pyomyositis, conjunctivitis, pneumonia, empyema, endocarditis, acute pericarditis, liver and spleen abscess, and primary cutaneous infection • Y pseudoturberculosis fever, scarlatiniform rash and abdominal symptoms • Pseudoappendiceal pain—ileocecal mesenteric adenitis or terminal ileitis • Can mimic Kawasaki disease
Clostridium difficile	• Antibiotic exposure • Contact with infected host or infected object	Watery diarrhea, abdominal pain, fever	Pseudomembranous colitis, toxic megacolon
Vibrio cholera	Contaminated food or water	Painless, copious watery diarrhea, colorless stools with flecks of mucus	Severe dehydration and electrolyte disturbance, coma, shock

is a 22% resistance rate to fluoroquinolones in children. Treatment course is generally 5 to 7 days.[6]

Patients with septicemia, immunocompromise, or sites of infection other than the GI tract with enterocolitis due to *Y enterocolitica* should receive antibiotics. Treatment can decrease the duration of fecal excretion and decrease symptoms. It is usually susceptible to TMP-SMX. Aminoglycosides, cefotaxime, fluoroquinolones, and doxycycline are additional options. Resistance to first-generation cephalosporins and most penicillins is typical.[7]

There are at least 5 types of *E coli* that produce diarrhea. However, enterohemorrhagic *E coli* is the type that commonly causes disease in the United States. Strains that produce Shiga-toxin (STEC) have been associated with hemolytic-uremic syndrome (HUS). Of these, STEC O157:H7 is the most virulent strain. HUS will occur in up to 20% of patients with STEC O157:H7 and up to 50% can require dialysis, with a 3% to 5% mortality rate. Thrombotic thrombocytopenic purpura occurs in adults. A meta-analysis did not show that children have a greater chance of developing HUS if treated with antibiotics for STEC. However, most experts still do not treat *E coli* O157:H7 with antibiotic therapy.[8]

The diarrhea caused by enteropathogenic *E coli* (EPEC) is generally found in developing countries and causes severe diarrhea that can lead to dehydration and death. Enteroinvasive *E coli* (EIEC) is similar in many ways to a *Shigella* infection. Enteroaggregative *E coli* (EAEC) can cause acute and chronic diarrhea in developed and underdeveloped countries. The enterotoxigenic *E coli* (ETEC) is uncommon in the United States but causes a moderate severity diarrhea in resource-limited countries and is the most common cause of traveler's diarrhea. For travelers' diarrhea, a course of azithromycin, or a fluoroquinolone in those older than 18 years, can be helpful. Other antimicrobial agents that may be used are TMP-SMX and doxycycline. A Cochrane review found that although there were more adverse events in those who took antibiotics for travelers' diarrhea, most of the side effects were minor and the patients benefited clinically from the therapy.[8]

C difficile is present as a colonizing organism in ~50% of infants younger than 1 year of age. Therefore, careful consideration should be undertaken before determining this bacterium as a pathogen. This organism causes a range of illness from mild antibiotic-associated diarrhea to severe pseudomembranous colitis with systemic toxicity, bloody diarrhea, and a tender abdomen. If the laboratory diagnosis is consistent with the history and clinical features, then treatment should begin with removing the offending antibiotic agent if one is present. Metronidazole is recommended for those with severe disease who do not recover with antibiotic removal. It can be given orally or intravenously. Vancomycin is a second-line agent used only for cases in which metronidazole is ineffective. Vancomycin is only effective when given orally or by rectal enema for *C difficile*. Therapy should be administered for at least 10 days and relapse is common. The same treatment can be given for a second course.[9]

V cholera should be treated with enteral or parenteral rehydration therapy first. For moderate to severe cases, antimicrobial therapy with doxycycline or tetracycline is generally helpful and may outweigh the risk of dental staining. Based on antibiotic resistance patterns, additional therapies may include ciprofloxacin, ofloxacin, or TMP-SMX. Azithromycin may also be beneficial as a therapy in children.[10]

References

1. Dennehy PH. Acute diarrheal disease in children: epidemiology, prevention, and treatment. *Infect Dis Clin North Am.* 2005;19(3):585-602.

2. Diniz-Santos DR, Silva LR, Silva N. Antibiotics for the empirical treatment of acute infectious diarrhea in children. *Braz J Infect Dis.* 2006;10(3);217-227.

3. De Bruyn G, Hahn S, Borwick A. Antibiotic treatment for travellers'diarrhoea. *Cochrane Database Syst Rev.* 2000;(3): CD002242. doi: 10.1002/14651858.CD002242

4. American Academy of Pediatrics. *Shigella* infections. In: Pickering LK, Baker CJ, Kimberlin DW, Long SS, eds. *Red Book: 2009 Report of the Committee on Infectious Diseases.* 28th ed. Elk Grove Village, IL: American Academy of Pediatrics; 2009:593-595.

5. American Academy of Pediatrics. *Salmonella* infections. In: Pickering LK, Baker CJ, Kimberlin DW, Long SS, eds. *Red Book: 2009 Report of the Committee on Infectious Diseases.* 28th ed. Elk Grove Village, IL: American Academy of Pediatrics; 2009: 584-589.

6. American Academy of Pediatrics. *Campylobacter* infections. In: Pickering LK, Baker CJ, Kimberlin DW, Long SS, eds. *Red Book: 2009 Report of the Committee on Infectious Diseases.* 28th ed. Elk Grove Village, IL:American Academy of Pediatrics; 2009:243-245.

7. American Academy of Pediatrics. *Yersinia enterocolitica* and *Yersinia pseudotuberculosis* infections. In: Pickering LK, Baker CJ, Kimberlin DW, Long SS, eds. *Red Book: 2009 Report of the Committee on Infectious Diseases.* 28th ed. Elk Grove Village, IL: American Academy of Pediatrics; 2009:733-735.

8. American Academy of Pediatrics. *Escherichia coli* diarrhea. In: Pickering LK, Baker CJ, Kimberlin DW, Long SS, eds. *Red Book: 2009 Report of the Committee on Infectious Diseases.* 28th ed. Elk Grove Village, IL: American Academy of Pediatrics; 2009:294-298.

9. American Academy of Pediatrics. *Clostridium difficile.* In: Pickering LK, Baker CJ, Kimberlin DW, Long SS, eds. *Red Book: 2009 Report of the Committee on Infectious Diseases.* 28th ed. Elk Grove Village, IL: American Academy of Pediatrics; 2009:257-265.

10. American Academy of Pediatrics. *Vibrio* infections. In: Pickering LK, Baker CJ, Kimberlin DW, Long SS, eds. *Red Book: 2009 Report of the Committee on Infectious Diseases.* 28th ed. Elk Grove Village, IL: American Academy of Pediatrics; 2009:727-729.

What Are Likely to Be the Most Common Viral Pathogens Causing Diarrhea Since the Decrease in Rotavirus Cases With Increase in Vaccine Uptake?

Amber Hoffman, MD

The answer to this question is currently evolving, but is being actively monitored. Diarrheal illnesses continue to be a leading cause of morbidity in US children, particularly for those younger than 5 years of age. Approximately 95% of children will experience a rotavirus infection by the time they are 5 years old, regardless of whether they live in a developed or developing country. The universality of rotavirus infection, coupled with its significant disease burden, made it a target for vaccine development. Rotavirus is the most common viral etiology for severe diarrhea in children under 5 years of age, and symptoms generally last for 3 to 8 days.[1] The other major viral pathogens responsible for acute gastroenteritis (AGE) are norovirus, astrovirus, and adenovirus.

Noroviruses (NoVs) belong to the Caliciviridae family and are the most common cause of AGE in the United States. Difficulty with detection of NoVs make them a challenge to study. They appear to be emerging and spreading according to a study that examined data regarding NoV outbreaks from 2001 to 2007 from 15 institutions on 5 continents. They are estimated to cause 23 million cases of AGE annually in the United States each year, and account for 90% of community outbreaks of viral AGE. NoV epidemic outbreaks continue to occur primarily in health care settings, military establishments, cruise ships, and schools. NoV infections peak in the winter, but off-season peaks in the spring or summer have occurred. Overall, the illness with NoV tends to be milder and shorter than rotavirus, lasting from 24 to 60 hours, and is typically characterized by the acute onset of nonbloody diarrhea, nausea, vomiting, and abdominal cramps. Some individuals may only manifest emesis and children may experience only mild-to-moderate diarrhea.[2]

Enteric adenovirus (EAd) infections occur throughout the year and primarily affect children younger than 4 years. The ones primarily associated with enteric disease are types 40, 41, and 31. They typically make up a smaller percentage of children admitted to the hospital for severe disease. In an Australian study that looked at AGE admissions to a teaching hospital from 1981 to 1992, EAd was identified by electron microscopy in only 3.4% of admissions as compared to rotavirus, which was found in 34.7%. In other studies involving hospitalized AGE, EAd infections caused between 1.1% and 7.9% of cases. Fluctuations in Ad41 prevalence, or antigenic changes of Ad41, may lead to increased infection rates as the proportion of susceptible individuals in the community is higher. In comparison with children admitted with rotavirus disease, those with EAd were more likely to have been sick for several days before admission with vomiting and diarrhea, but less likely to have been highly febrile or dehydrated. The mean number of symptomatic days was 9 in this study.[3]

Astrovirus infections are generally characterized by a short period of diarrhea along with vomiting, fever, and some abdominal pain. Symptoms generally last 5 to 6 days and are associated with mild dehydration, although asymptomatic infections can also occur. Children younger than 4 years of age are mainly affected, and the peak is in late winter and early spring. They have been detected in up to 10% to 34% of sporadic cases of community viral diarrhea but are responsible for a much lower number of severe cases causing hospitalization. The incidence of astroviruses causing AGE ranges from 2% to 9% in both developing and developed countries. In a 2004–2005 study of outpatient visits in China, 9.87% of children younger than 3 years had astrovirus by polymerase chain reaction (PCR).[4] A Barcelona study conducted between 1997 and 2000 identified astrovirus in 4.9% of cases, with coinfection in 17.2%. Of those that identified astrovirus, only 34.6% required admission, and 13.5% of infections were identified as nosocomial infections.[5]

Prior to the implementation of the rotavirus vaccines RotaTeq (Merck and Company; Whitehouse Station, New Jersey] [RV5]) and Rotarix (GlaxoSmithKline Biologicals; Rixensart, Belgium [RV1]), Taiwan evaluated the epidemiology of viral gastroenteritis between spring 2004 and 2006 by PCR testing. Six point three percent of the total number of AGE cases were sampled and 81.7% were virus positive. Rotavirus was found in 30.4% of samples, norovirus 19.8%, astrovirus 2.7%, and adenovirus 19.8%. Mixed infections were found in 20.3%. Of the mixed infections, 85% were rotavirus positive, making it the most common viral etiology of hospitalized AGE in this region.[6]

The Centers for Disease Control and Prevention New Vaccine Surveillance Network began population-based surveillance of AGE after RV5 was licensed and recommended by the Advisory Committee on Immunization Practices for routine immunization of infants in February 2006.[7] The system was designed to estimate disease burden of rotavirus as well as the impact of vaccination. RV1 was then recommended in June 2008. When evaluating the impact of rotavirus vaccination on the epidemiology of other viral AGE, it is helpful to understand these 2 vaccines.

Rotaviruses are classified based on their outer capsid proteins—G protein and P protein. These proteins are critical to vaccine development because they are targets for antibodies. Common US strains are P[8]G1, P[4]G2, P[8]G3, P[8]G4, P[8]G9, and P[6]G9, but there have been more than 40 different strains identified in the United States and globally. RV5 is a live, oral, human-bovine reassortment rotavirus vaccine that expresses the outer capsid proteins of 5 common strains (G1, G2, G3, G4, and P[8]G9 subgroup P1A) and showed a high level of efficacy against G1-G4 and G9 serotypes in the Rotavirus Efficacy and Safety Trial (REST).[1] During that study period, however, there were only 14% non-G1 strains in circulation. In a 3-year follow-up of Finnish children who were a part of REST, there was an 82% efficacy against the P[4]G2 strain. RV1 is a monovalent P[8]G1 vaccine, and in a Latin American and Finnish trial had an efficacy of 82% to 96% against severe rotavirus disease.[8]

It is difficult to determine now whether strain-specific variations are related to vaccination or natural shift, and whether that possible antigenic shift, or drift, will impact the predominance of strains against which current vaccines do not confer immunity. This may impact whether other viruses responsible for AGE will predominate.[9] From January through April 2008, which was approximately 2 years after US licensure of RotaTeq, there was a 79% decline in rotavirus detection when compared with 15 years of previous data. There was also a 90% decrease in severe rotavirus visits to the hospital, emergency department, and outpatient clinics in a population-based study when compared with previous years. This study did not look at the incidence of other viral pathogens in those seen with AGE who did not test positive for rotavirus.[10]

The National Respiratory and Enteric Virus Surveillance System (NREVSS) is a network of 67 laboratories across the United States that report rotavirus positivity. Data from NREVSS was analyzed during the 2007 to 2008 rotavirus season and compared with the prevaccine seasons from 2000 to 2006. In the prevaccination period, the median peak in rotavirus activity in the United States occurred in early March with 44% of specimens returning positive for rotavirus.[11] In 2007 to 2008, it peaked in late April with 17% of specimens testing positive. Overall, the entire rotavirus season was delayed for each region of the country studied, and there were fewer cases, but the season ended at the same time as it had in the prevaccination era in mid-June, resulting in a season that was approximately 2 weeks shorter. The national immunization rate in December 2007 among infants age 3 months having received 1 rotavirus vaccine was 58%. Although the rotavirus season was delayed, shorter in duration, and diminished in the magnitude of disease burden, the changes seemed greater than what can be explained by vaccination rates alone. There may be indirect benefits such as herd immunity.[12] In addition, hospitalization rates have also been evaluated in 18 US states comparing prevaccine 2000 to 2006 median rate with the postvaccine timeframes, with a finding that overall there was a 16% reduction in hospitalizations in 2007 and a 46% reduction by 2008 across all age groups.[13] In a Mexican study, diarrhea-related deaths decreased by 35% in children younger than 5 years and 41% in children who were 11 months or younger after 74% of children 11 months or under received 1 dose of rotavirus vaccine.[14]

Although both rotavirus vaccines have clearly been shown to be effective in the decreasing hospitalization rates due to rotavirus, it remains to be seen how much of a role serotype switching will play in the future of childhood diarrheal diseases. Therefore, the answer to the question regarding the changing epidemiology of viral causes of AGE is complicated due to the changing epidemiology of the 4 most common viruses as well as their own antigenic changes. Continued surveillance to follow the trends of immunization rates, serotype predominance, and incidence of other viral causes of AGE will hopefully provide a more definitive answer to this question in the future.

References

1. Payne DC, Stockman LJ, Gentsch JR, Parashar UD. *Rotavirus.* Centers for Disease Control and Prevention. In: Manual for the Surveillance of Vaccine-Preventable Diseases. 4th Edition, 2008-2009 & 5th Edition, 2011.
2. Siebenga JJ, Vennema H, Zheng DP, et al. Norovirus illness is a global problem: emergence and spread of norovirus GII.4 varients, 2001-2007. *J Infect Dis.* 2009;200(5):802-812.
3. Grimwood K. Patients with enteric adenovirus gastroenteritis admitted to an Australian pediatric teaching hospital from 1981-1992. *J Clin Microbiol.* 1995;33:131-136.
4. Liu MQ, Yang B-F, Peng J-S, et al. Molecular epidemiology of astrovirus infection in infants in Wuhan, China. *J Clin Microbiol.* 2007;45(4):1308-1309.
5. Guix S, Santiago C, Villena C, et al. Molecular epidemiology of astrovirus infection in Barcelona, Spain. *J Clin Microbiol.* 2002;40(1):133-139.
6. Chen SY, Chang Y-U, Lee Y-S, et al. Molecular epidemiology and clinical manifestations of viral gastroenteritis in hospitalized pediatric patients in Northern Taiwan. *J Clin Microbiol.* 2007;45(6):2054-2057.
7. Payne DC, Staat MA, Edwards KM, et al. Active, population-based surveillance for severe rotavirus gastroenteritis in children in the United States. *Pediatrics.* 2008;112(6):1235-1243.
8. Patel MM, Parashar UD. Assessing the effectiveness and public health impact of rotavirus vaccines after introduction in immunization programs. *J Infect Dis.* 2009:200(suppl 1):S291-S298.
9. O'Ryan M. The ever-changing landscape of rotavirus serotypes. *Pediatr Infect Dis J.* 2009;28(3 suppl):S60-S62.
10. Payne DC, Parashar UD. Epidemiological shifts in severe acute gastroenteritis in US children: will rotavirus vaccination change the picture? *J Pediatr.* 2008;153(6):737-738.
11. Payne DC, Szilagyi PG, Staat MA, et al. Secular variation in United States rotavirus disease rates and serotypes. *Pediatr Infect Dis J.* 2009;28(11):948-953.
12. Tate JE, Panozzo CA, Payne DC, et al. Decline and change in seasonality of US rotavirus activity after the introduction of rotavirus vaccine. *Pediatrics.* 2009;124(2):465-471.
13. Curns AT, Steiner CA, Barrett M, Hunter K, Wilson E, Parashar UD. Reduction in acute gastroenteriris hospitalizations among US children after introduction of rotavirus vaccine: analysis of hospital discharge data from 18 US states. *J Infect Dis.* 2010;201(11):1617-1624.
14. Richardson V, Hernandez-Pichardo J, Quintanar-Solares M, et al. Effect of rotavirus vaccination on death from childhood diarrhea in Mexico. *N Engl J Med.* 2010;362(4):299-305.

SECTION X

UPPER RESPIRATORY TRACT INFECTION/SINUSITIS

33

WHEN SHOULD I BE WORRIED ABOUT IMMUNE DEFICIENCY IN THE SETTING OF RECURRENT UPPER RESPIRATORY TRACT INFECTIONS?

Adam L. Hersh, MD, PhD

It is not unusual for immunocompetent children to have 6 to 8 self-limited upper respiratory tract infections (URIs) or "colds" per year; children in day care or those with older siblings may experience even more frequent infections. Likewise, recurrent otitis media is common in healthy children. Predisposing factors to recurrent URIs and otitis media include allergies, passive exposure to cigarette smoke, anatomical defects of the upper or lower airway, and even gastroesophageal reflux. However, recurrent URIs can sometimes be the presenting sign of a more serious underlying immune defect, which limits the capacity of the patient to mount effective immune responses.

Host defense against microbes (eg, viruses, bacteria, and fungi) are the result of a complex network of cells capable of recognizing a broad array of pathogens. The immune system can be broadly divided into 2 categories: innate and adaptive immunity. Innate immune cells are found in relative abundance throughout the body and include neutrophils, basophils, mast cells, eosinophils, monocytes, macrophages, and dendritic cells. The adaptive immune system includes T and B lymphocytes. These cells express a cell-surface receptor (the T-cell or B-cell receptor). Through a complex developmental process, these receptors allow relatively rare cells to recognize a specific infection and respond accordingly. The amplification of T- and B-cell populations is the basis of the generation of protective immunity from vaccination. Typically, patients who have immune deficiency in the setting of recurrent URIs have deficiencies in adaptive immunity. In particular, dysfunction in either B or T cells leads to poor antibody production (or quality) and subsequent susceptibility to sinopulmonary infections. Most commonly, these humoral immune deficiencies lead to recurrent infection with encapsulated organisms, including *Streptococcus pneumonia* and *Haemophilus influenzae*. Antibody production disorders can have varied levels of T-cell dysfunction that may place the patient at increased risk for severe viral or opportunistic infections as well. Humoral immune deficiencies that might present with recurrent URIs include X-linked agammaglobulinemia, common variable immuno-deficiency (CVID), selective immunoglobulin (Ig)A deficiency, polysaccharide antibody deficiency with or without IgG subclass deficiency, and hyper IgM syndrome (with the X-linked being the most severe because of T-cell dysfunction). Of these, CVID and selective IgA deficiency would be the highest consideration in a patient with recurrent URIs as these 2 disorders are most prevalent. Transient hypogammaglobulinemia of infancy should also be considered in young children. Other immune deficiencies that have been associated with recurrent URIs, including otitis media, human immunodeficiency virus infection, DiGeorge syndrome, and Wiskott-Aldrich syndrome.

When a patient presents with recurrent URIs, the clinical history is the starting point. Increased frequency or severity of infections or infections with unusual organisms should raise suspicion of immune deficiency, as should episodes of otitis media or sinusitis that fail to respond to oral antibiotics. Frequent URIs seen in the context of other frequent infections such as pneumonia or meningitis are another red flag. If a patient has 4 or more distinct episodes of severe (does not respond with typical therapy or requires repeated parenteral therapy) otitis media or 2 or more episodes of pneumonia/sinusitis in 1 year, immunodeficiency should at least be considered. A family history of severe infections requiring courses of antibiotics and/or hospitalization also raises concern.

Screening tests for suspected humoral immune deficiency include a complete blood count, quantitative serum immunoglobulins (IgG, IgA, IgM, quantitative IgG subclasses), IgG levels to specific protein vaccine antigens such as diphtheria or tetanus, and HIV anti-body. When indicated by clinical examination or abnormalities in screening laboratories, lymphocyte subset analysis to document appropriate numbers and proportions of B and T cells might also be performed.

If consideration of allergic rhinitis as a cause of frequent or recurrent sinopulmonary infections is being given, then referral to an allergist may be helpful. However, if there is significant concern that the child in fact has recurrent infections that are out of the norm for his or her age group, then referral to an immunologist or an infectious diseases specialist may be warranted for further diagnostic testing and treatment strategies.

Suggested Readings

American Academy of Pediatrics Subcommittee on Management of Acute Otitis Media. Diagnosis and management of acute otitis media. *Pediatrics.* 2004;113(5): 1451–1465.

Ballow M. Approach to the patient with recurrent infections. *Clin Rev AllergImmunol.* 2008;34(2):129-140.

Bonilla FA, Bernstein IL, Khan DA, et al. Practice parameter for the diagnosis and management of primary immuno-deficiency. *Ann Allergy Astham Immun.* 2005;94(5 suppl 1):S1-S63.

Long SS, Pickering LK, Prober CG, eds. *Principles and Practice of Pediatric Infectious Diseases.* 3rd ed. Philadelphia, PA: Churchill Livingston/Elsevier; 2009.

Wilson NW, Hogan MB. Otitis media as presenting complaint in childhood immunodeficiency diseases. *Curr Allergy Asthma Rep.* 2008,8(6):519-524.

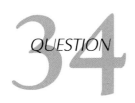
WHAT ARE THE MOST COMMON VIRAL RESPIRATORY PATHOGENS IN INFANTS IN THE FIRST YEAR OF LIFE?

Adam L. Hersh, MD, PhD

Viral respiratory infections are an inevitable fact during the first year of life for infants. Numerous prospective studies have estimated that on average, infants experience 3 to 8 viral respiratory infections during their first year. These infections vary widely in their severity. Although most are mild and self-limited, some episodes are severe, requiring hospitalization, which occurs in approximately 3% of children under the age of 1 year on an annual basis in the United States.

The etiology of the viral pathogens causing respiratory infections for infants is well established. With the advent of newer molecular-based diagnostic technology, the ability to identify a causative pathogen for viral respiratory infections is greatly enhanced. The 2 most frequently isolated pathogens are respiratory syncytial virus (RSV) and human rhinovirus. Other important viral pathogens include enterovirus; influenza A and B viruses; human metapneumovirus (hMPV); adenovirus; and parainfluenza 1, 2, and 3 viruses. Additionally, bocavirus has been recently discovered, and its relative importance in causation and severity of viral illness is currently being evaluated. Certain viruses follow well-established seasonal patterns such as influenza and RSV, with peak activity during winter months in temperate climates, whereas others may have sporadic activity throughout the year (eg, adenovirus, rhinovirus). There is a classic sequence of respiratory viral appearance in communities after children return to school in the fall of the year in temperate climates. The first seasonal virus to appear is usually parainfluenza causing croup in September–October, followed soon after by the appearance of RSV. RSV peaks generally around December through January but persists through April. In Florida, RSV season is longer. Influenza generally appears in late December and continues through the spring of the year—cocirculating with RSV. There may be a second parainfluenza season in late spring as influenza and RSV wane (Table 34-1).

Table 34-1
Common Viruses, Symptoms and Seasonality Among Infants

Virus	Symptoms	Season (Peak)
Influenza A and B	Fever, prostration, malaise, myalgias, headache, cough, sore throat, congestion, rhinitis	November through May (January/ February)
RSV	URI, cough, wheezing, tachypnea, apnea, respiratory distress	November through March and into April east of the Mississippi river (December/January/February)
Adenovirus	URI, otitis media, pharyngitis, tonsillitis, bronchiolitis, pneumonia, pharyngoconjunctival fever, gastroenteritis	Throughout year (late spring/ early summer)
Rhinovirus	URI, pharyngitis, otitis media, bronchiolitis, pneumonia	Throughout year (fall/spring)
Parainfluenza 1, 2, 3	Laryngotracheobronchitis (croup), URI, bronchiolitis, pneumonia	Type 1—Outbreaks of croup every other year in autumn Type 2—Outbreaks of URI/croup occur with type 1, but less severe and less common Type 3—Prominent cause of LRI in spring/summer/early fall
Enterovirus	Undifferentiated febrile illness, URI/LRI, exanthema, gastrointestinal/ genitourinary symptomatology, myositis, conjunctivitis, myocarditis	June through October (August)
Bocavirus	Fever, URI, wheezing	Throughout year (spring)
hMPV	Bronchiolitis, pneumonia, croup, URI, otitis media, asthma exacerbations	Sporadic infection throughout year (late winter/early spring, coinciding with RSV)

LRI = lower respiratory infection; RSV = respiratory syncytial virus; URI = upper respiratory infection

Because of overlap in respiratory viral seasons, coinfections can occur. Coinfection with more than 1 viral pathogen is common, occurring in 16% to 47% of hospitalized children, although most estimates are ~20%. The most common organism in this setting is RSV with another coinfecting pathogen. The data on whether having more than one viral pathogen simultaneously confers more severe disease are conflicting, with some studies showing no difference and others showing higher hospitalization and intensive care unit admission rates. A recent study from Brazil compared infants younger than 1 year with confirmed RSV to those with RSV and another viral pathogen, with adenovirus and hMPV being the most common coinfecting organisms. The authors compared the

2 groups on 4 severity factors (ie, total length of hospitalization, duration of oxygen therapy, admission to the intensive care unit, and need for mechanical ventilation) and found no difference in those infants with RSV alone versus RSV with a coinfecting pathogen. Another study from the UK compared infants younger than 2 years of age with RSV alone and RSV with hMPV coinfection and found that coinfected infants had a 10-fold increase in risk of intensive care unit admission. However, there was no association found with dual infection and severe disease compared to having moderate disease.

Among the previously mentioned viruses, RSV is the most frequently identified virus in the young child regardless of clinical severity. RSV is also the most common cause of bronchiolitis, detected in 43% to 74% of cases. Bronchiolitis is a condition characterized by acute inflammation, cellular necrosis, edema, and increased mucous production, which in turn causes airway obstruction particularly in the smallest terminal bronchioles, and associated air trapping (hyperinflation) and wheezing. Infants may manifest with hypoxia, tachypnea, retractions, and a need for frequent suctioning. RSV is among the leading causes of hospitalization for children under the age of 2 and is the direct cause in >120,000 hospitalizations annually in children younger than 1 year in the United States. Clinical factors placing infants at particularly high risk for hospitalization with RSV include chronic lung disease, prematurity, neurologic impairment, and congenital heart disease. Although treatment options for this infection are mainly supportive in nature, prevention with palivizumab (Synagis, a humanized mouse monoclonal antibody) is recommended for certain high-risk hosts during the first, and sometimes the second, RSV season.

It was previously believed that the clinical spectrum of disease caused by rhinovirus was limited to the common cold and upper respiratory tract infections. More recently, using molecular-based diagnostic technology, rhinovirus has been identified as among the most commonly identified organisms in community-acquired lower respiratory tract infections in children and thus is suspected to play an important role in these infections as well.

The clinician should consider what it is he or she will do with the result of the test prior to embarking on an attempt to diagnose a certain viral pathogen. In the patient who is clinically well appearing with only mild upper respiratory infection/lower respiratory infection (URI/LRI) symptoms, the cost of diagnostic testing and the discomfort of the child from either nasal swab or deeper nasopharyngeal suction may not make this a worthwhile endeavor. However, establishing a diagnosis of a viral etiology via diagnostic testing, in certain instances, has important clinical utility. Testing is useful for surveillance and establishing that certain viruses are circulating, even in the office setting. It allows the clinician to provide anticipatory guidance to families regarding the possibility of development of further symptomatology, communicability, and the expected length of illness, especially in the setting of coinfecting organisms. Confirming a diagnosis of influenza is also probably the most frequently clinically useful, especially among patients at high risk for complications, because early antiviral treatment is beneficial and is recommended. Furthermore, establishing a viral diagnosis may assist in efforts to prescribe antibiotics judiciously, as in certain instances this reduces (or eliminates) the possibility of a bacterial infection.

Suggested Readings

American Academy of Pediatrics Subcommittee on Management of Acute Otitis Media. Diagnosis and management of acute otitis media. *Pediatrics*. 2004;113(5):1451-1465.

De Paulis M, Gilio AE, Ferraro AA, et al. Severity of viral coinfection in hospitalized infants with respiratory syncytial virus infection. *J Pediatr (Rio J)*. 2011;87(4):307-313.

Long SS, Pickering LK, Prober CG, eds. *Principles and Practice of Pediatric Infectious Diseases*, 3rd ed. Philadelphia, PA: Churchill Livingston/Elsevier; 2009.

Pavia A. Viral infections of the lower respiratory tract: old viruses, new viruses, and the role of diagnosis. *CID*. 2011;52:S284-S289.

Semple MG, Cowell A, Dove W, et al. Dual infection of infants by human metapneumovirus and human respiratory syncytial virus is strongly associated with severe bronchiolitis. *J Infect Dis*. 2005;191(3):382-386.

Tregoning JS, Schwarze J. Respiratory viral infections in infants: causes, clinical symptoms, virology and immunology. *Clin Microbiol Rev*. 2010;23(1):74-98.

Van Woensel JB, Aalderen WM, Kimpen JL. Viral lower respiratory tract infection in infants and young children. *BMJ*. 2003;327(7405):36-40.

WHAT ANTIBIOTICS ARE RECOMMENDED EMPIRICALLY FOR ACUTE BACTERIAL SINUSITIS IN A PATIENT WHO HAS NOT RECEIVED ANTIBIOTICS RECENTLY?

Adam L. Hersh, MD, PhD

The American Academy of Pediatrics currently recommends amoxicillin as the first-line empiric antibiotic for acute bacterial sinusitis. Whether or not to use standard dose (45 mg/kg/day) versus high dose (80 to 90 mg/kg/day) depends on the prevalence of penicillin nonsusceptible *Streptococcus pneumoniae* in your community, and whether the strains are high versus intermediate in their resistance level. Although there is no definitive recommendation, many experts suggest using high-dose amoxicillin if the prevalence of high penicillin resistance (mean inhibitory concentration [MIC] >1.0 mg/L) exceeds 15% to 20%.

The rationale for recommending amoxicillin is that *S pneumoniae* is the most common and the most clinically important pathogen causing acute bacterial sinusitis in children. Amoxicillin in high doses effectively treats most (up to 90%) penicillin non-susceptible strains of *S pneumoniae* in most communities (up to MICs of 4.0 mg/L as extrapolated from acute otitis media [AOM] studies). This is because the mechanism of action for penicillin (also applies to amoxicillin) resistance occurs by alteration in penicillin-binding proteins (PBPs). Although altered PBPs have reduced affinity for the antibiotic, this lower affinity is largely overcome via higher doses of the drug, as there is more drug present in the vicinity of the bacteria (see Question 19 for a more detailed explanation).

The first-line treatment recommendation in some guidelines is amoxicillin-clavulanate, especially for those children who are at higher risk for complications (eg, severe symptoms at presentation) or a drug-resistant pathogen (eg, recent amoxicillin exposure or day care attendance). It is important to note that this should be accomplished using a high dose of the amoxicillin component without doubling the dose of the beta-lactamase inhibitor, as higher doses of clavulanate are known to cause more severe diarrhea. Formulations of amoxicillin-clavulanate with 400 mg/5 mL of amoxicillin have the desired proportions of clavulanate to minimize gastrointestinal adverse effects. Additionally, there is no added therapeutic benefit to higher doses of clavulanate. The rationale for high-dose amoxicillin with standard-dose clavulanate is based on the fact that patients with acute bacterial sinusitis could have a highly resistant strain of *S pneumoniae*, or another pathogen that is penicillin resistant by virtue of beta-lactamase production, such as nontypeable *Haemophilus influenzae* and *Moraxella catarrhalis*. Because the prevalence of these organisms among patients with acute bacterial sinusitis (and AOM) appears to be increasing (especially for *H influenzae*), some experts advocate initiating therapy with amoxicillin-clavulanate as the first-line therapy for all patients, especially in communities where the prevalence of *H influenzae* is known to be high. Community and regional differences in prevalence of these organisms underscore the importance of the clinician having knowledge of his or her local pathogens and resistance patterns. Remember that no pneumococcus has ever produced beta-lactamase, so use of clavulanate in this instance does not increase efficacy against pneumococcus, but does extend the efficacy of amoxicillin to include beta-lactamase producing nontypeable *H influenzae* and *M catarrhalis*, methicillin-sensitive *Staphylococcus aureus* (MSSA), and selected anaerobes.

It is important to remember that in the patient who is not showing clinical improvement or is clinically worsening, complicated infection should be considered in addition to the possibility of resistant pathogens noted above. Common and or severe complications of bacterial sinusitis include orbital cellulitis and/or abscess, optic neuritis, Pott puffy tumor (frontal osteitis), sinus thrombosis, sub- or epidural empyema, brain abscess, or meningitis. At times, 1 or more of these complications occurs in an older patient with severe headache that develops over days to a week. Other pathogens must be considered in this setting including *S aureus* (including methicillin-resistant *Staphylococcus aureus* [MRSA]), *Streptococcus mitis*, *Fusobacterium necrophorum*, and other oral anaerobes. Some of these pathogens may be treated by the therapies mentioned above. However, a surgical approach may be necessary if 1 of the aforementioned complications has occurred, as obtaining a pathogen in this setting allows for more directed antibiotic therapy. In addition, surgical drainage has been shown to hasten recovery.

The introduction of the 7-valent pneumococcal conjugate vaccine (PCV) is at least partially responsible for the change in epidemiology that has shown an increase in beta-lactamase producing nontypeable *H influenzae* and highly penicillin resistant type 19A pneumococcus. Many of the serotypes of *S pneumoniae* that were previously common causes of sinusitis have been eliminated by use of PCV7 and we will likely see similar reduction in the added 6 serotypes in recently released 13-valent PCV. This recent use of 13-valent PCV should in particular reduce the prevalence of type 19A pneumococcus by 2012, but beta-lactamase producing nontypeable *H influenzae* will likely remain very common. Revised treatment guidelines from the American Academy of Pediatrics and the Infectious Diseases Society of America are currently under development and will address this issue. Until they are available, the antibiotic treatment choices as to other specific drugs (eg, in cases with penicillin allergy) parallel that of AOM (see the questions on AOM for more details). Keep your eyes open for these new guidelines because recommendations may change.

Suggested Readings

American Academy of Pediatrics. Subcommittee on Management of Sinusitis and Committee on Quality Improvement. Clinical practice guideline: management of sinusitis. *Pediatrics*. 2001;108(3):798-808.

Anon JB, Jacobs MR, Poole MD, Singer ME. First-line vs second-line antibiotics for treatment of sinusitis. *JAMA*. 2002;287(11):1395-1396.

Meltzer EO, Hamilos DL. Rhinosinusitis diagnosis and management for the clinician: a synopsis of recent consensus guidelines. *Mayo Clin Proc*. 2011;86(5):427-443.

National guidelines for use of imaging in diagnosis of acute sinusitis: http://www.guidelines.gov/content.aspx?id=1 5752&search=Acute+sinusitis

Taylor A, Adam HM. Sinusitis. *Pediatr Rev*. 2006;27(10):395-397.

36

WHAT ANTIBIOTICS ARE RECOMMENDED TO TREAT ACUTE BACTERIAL SINUSITIS IN THE PATIENT WHO HAD A COURSE OF AMOXICILLIN WITHIN THE LAST FEW WEEKS FOR OTITIS MEDIA?

Adam L. Hersh, MD, PhD

There are several possibilities that could explain the subsequent development of acute sinusitis after treatment with amoxicillin for acute otitis media (AOM). From a microbiologic standpoint, the expected bacterial causes of acute sinusitis and AOM are known to be identical and so the recommended antibiotic therapy is similar. Thus, in this instance, the clinician must first be confident in the diagnosis of acute bacterial sinusitis because alternative diagnoses such as a viral upper respiratory infection (URI), which has similar symptoms to acute bacterial sinusitis, may be the actual cause of the infection. See the recent American Academy of Pediatrics (AAP) guidelines edited by Dr. Ellen Wald[1] on the diagnosis of acute bacterial sinusitis. Note that green or yellow drainage occurs with nearly every viral URI (usually on day 3 to 5 of drainage) and is not pathognomic or even highly suggestive of acute bacterial sinusitis. The discoloration of nasal drainage with viral URIs is due to increased cellular elements, including monocytes, macrophages, as well as neutrophils together with debris from injured or sloughed respiratory epithelium. Another noninfectious condition such as allergy is also very common and can present in a similar fashion. In the case of allergy, more detailed aspects of the patient history and additional symptoms such as itching in the nose or eyes may be a clue.

If the diagnostic certainty for acute bacterial sinusitis is high (eg, symptoms exceeding 10 days, or increasing in intensity after day 7 plus headache or facial or maxillary tooth pain), it is important to confirm that the duration and dosing of the prior amoxicillin was appropriate because inadequate treatment for AOM could predispose to subsequent sinusitis. This may occur if a persistent infection of the posterior nasopharynx occurs in the face of incompletely or inadequately treated AOM.

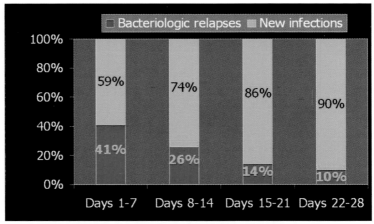

Figure 36-1. Proportion of AOM infections representing relapses versus new infections over time.

Another possible issue is whether the ostiomeatal complex became dysfunctional despite adequate AOM therapy during which the middle ear infection resolved. In other words, even though the initial infection was eradicated during the course of therapy, the sinuses may be unable to flush adequately and will become infected due to a mechanical problem. In this case, one may still select for amoxicillin resistance in the nasopharyngeal flora, which then enter the sinuses and cause infection. This has been well described for recurrent AOM, where Dagan et al[2] showed that the longer the interval between episodes, the more likely the cause of a subsequent episode is a new pathogen. For example, if a recurrence occurs at 7 days, the chance that the original pathogen is the cause is approximately 40%; this decreases to 25% after 2 weeks, 15% after 3 weeks, and 10% if 4 weeks has elapsed between episodes (Figure 36-1).

In this context whereby one is considering the diagnosis of sinusitis following a recent episode of AOM, one must be concerned that the prior amoxicillin therapy has selected for a different pathogen including a highly penicillin-resistant pneumococcus or a beta-lactamase-producing pathogen such as nontypeable *Haemophilus influenzae*. In this case, using a beta-lactamase stable drug with as much pneumococcal activity as possible is the goal. High-dose amoxicillin plus clavulanate is an ideal choice as high-dose amoxicillin provides good coverage even for resistant strains of pneumococcus, and the clavulanate adds coverage for beta-lactamase-producing *H influenzae* and *Moraxella catarrhalis*. Both amoxicillin and amoxicillin with clavulanate are readily available at most pharmacies, come in several concentrations, and are palatable. Other second-line alternatives to consider, especially in the case of penicillin allergy, include an oral third-generation cephalosporin, clindamycin, and azithromycin.[1] Some clinicians ask, "What is the highest dose of amoxicillin that can be used?" My answer is 100 mg/kg/day or up to 4 g/day of amoxicillin. Although this is not technically Food and Drug Administration approved as a sole product, this dose is FDA approved for Augmentin XR (GlaxoSmithKline Biologicals; Rixensart, Belgium). If the pharmacist questions your prescribing 4 g/day, you can refer him or her to the package insert for Augmentin XR.

The optimal duration of therapy for acute sinusitis is not well established, but 10 days has been effective in several clinical trials. There are data in adult-based studies that have shown effective treatment in as little as 3 days. However, this has not been established in children.

References

1. American Academy of Pediatrics Subcommittee on Management of Acute Otitis Media. Diagnosis and management of acute otitis media. *Pediatrics*. 2004;113(5):1451-1465.
2. Leibovitz E, Greenberg D, Piglansky L. Recurrent acute otitis media occurring within one month from completion of antibiotic therapy: relationship to the original pathogen. *Pediatr Infect Dis J*. 2003;22(3):209-216.

Suggested Reading

Leibovitz E, Greenberg D, Piglansky L, et al. Recurrent acute otitis media occurring within one month from completion of antibiotic therapy: relationship to the original pathogen. *Pediatr Infect Dis J*. 2003;22(3):209-216 (ISSN: 0891-3668).

SECTION XI

COMMUNITY-ACQUIRED PNEUMONIA

WHAT IS THE MOST COMMON PATHOGEN INVOLVED IN COMMUNITY-ACQUIRED PNEUMONIA, AND THE EMPIRIC THERAPY OF CHOICE IN THE PRESCHOOL–AGED CHILD WITH FEVER TO 102°F, RALES, AND A LOBAR INFILTRATE ON CHEST RADIOGRAPH?

Christopher R. Cannavino, MD

The etiologic agents of community-acquired pneumonia (CAP) vary by age and presenting signs and symptoms. Viral pathogens are far more common than bacterial pathogens as agents of CAP in children, particularly in the preschool–aged population. However, given a clinical presentation of high fever, rales, and a focal infiltrate on chest radiograph, typical bacterial CAP pathogens are most likely. Although the advent of polysaccharide–protein conjugate vaccines has altered the epidemiology of bacterial CAP, *Streptococcus pneumoniae* remains the most common cause, with strains demonstrating far less penicillin resistance than those isolated prior to widespread use of the pneumococcal conjugate vaccine. Amoxicillin is the first-line agent for oral empiric therapy in the outpatient setting as it provides adequate coverage for most pneumococcal isolates. A familiarity with the common pathogens and treatment regimens of CAP is important given the prevalence of disease in children and the potential for significant morbidity and mortality.

CAP is a common infection in the pediatric population, particularly in preschool–aged children. Children younger than 5 years old have an estimated annual incidence of 36 to 40 cases per 1000 children per year (versus 11 to 16 cases in children 5 to 14 years of age). The pathogens associated with CAP may be divided into 3 major groups: viral, atypical bacterial, and bacterial. In preschool–aged children, viral pathogens are the most common cause of CAP. Children with viral pneumonias tend to have less significant fever; diffuse, bilateral crackles on examination; and interstitial, perihilar bilateral infiltrates on chest radiographs. Atypical pneumonia-associated pathogens, such as *Chlamydophila pneumoniae* and *Mycoplasma pneumoniae*, are relatively uncommon in preschool–aged children. Children with atypical bacterial pneumonias tend to have low-grade fevers; nonfocal crackles and/or wheezing on examination; and bilateral patchy, reticulonodular infiltrates on chest radiographs. Although it should be noted that *M pneumoniae* may occasionally present with focal lobar infiltrates, this pathogen is seen primarily in children younger than 5 years old. Children with typical bacterial pneumonia tend to have significant fever, focal rales on examination, and unilateral segmental or lobar consolidations on chest radiographs. Thus, in the preschool–aged child with a clinical presentation similar to that in the vignette, bacterial pathogens are most likely.

S pneumoniae is the most common cause of bacterial CAP. Other typical bacterial causes of CAP include *Haemophilus influenzae*, *Staphylococcus aureus*, and *Streptococcus pyogenes*. The widespread use of *H influenzae* type B conjugate vaccine has dramatically reduced the incidence of this pathogen in CAP. Nontype B or nontypable *H influenzae* strains may cause pneumonia, but they are less common than pneumococcal pneumonia. *S aureus* (including methicillin-resistant *S aureus*) is an uncommon, but important cause of CAP. Children with *S aureus* typically present with severe, rapidly progressive symptoms and often have features of complicated pneumonia. *S pyogenes* typically affects the upper respiratory tract, but occasionally is a cause of pneumonia. Although these pathogens are significant causes of bacterial CAP, *S pneumoniae* is the predominate pathogen in children. A study investigating the etiology of CAP in otherwise healthy hospitalized children found typical bacterial pathogens in 60% of cases, of which 73% were *S pneumoniae*.

S pneumoniae are gram-positive, catalase-negative, lancet-shaped diplococci. Rates of nasopharyngeal colonization in children may be extremely high. Transmission occurs via respiratory droplets. Serotypes of *S pneumoniae* are classified based on their polysaccharide capsule. The heptavalent pneumococcal conjugate vaccine (PCV7) targeted the most invasive and antibiotic-resistant serotypes in the United States. Prior to the widespread use of PCV7, these serotypes accounted for the majority of pneumococcal pneumonia. However, in the post-PCV7 era, serotype 19A emerged as the most common cause of invasive pneumococcal disease. Recently, a 13-valent conjugate vaccine (PCV13), which includes serotype 19A, was licensed in the United States. Although the impact of this expanded vaccine remains to be seen, at least 90 different pneumococcal serotypes exist and other serotypes may emerge in response to vaccine-induced selective pressure. Although the *S pneumoniae* conjugate vaccine has decreased the prevalence of vaccine-associated serotypes, pneumococcus remains the most common cause of bacterial CAP. Further, pneumococcal pneumonia has a high rate of complications (eg, parapneumonic effusions, empyemas) associated with significant morbidity and mortality. Thus, given the prevalence of disease in the pediatric population, recognition of the pathogens associated with bacterial CAP and appropriate treatment are essential.

Amoxicillin is the empiric oral antimicrobial therapy of choice for children with suspected bacterial CAP. Amoxicillin is well tolerated and provides good coverage for the vast majority of *S pneumoniae* isolates. Historically, amoxicillin was dosed at 40 to 45 mg/kg/d divided 3 times per day. This "standard dose" achieved concentrations that provided sufficient time above the minimum inhibitory concentration to eradicate highly susceptible pneumococci. However, with the emergence of penicillin-nonsusceptible *S pneumoniae* in the 1990s, "high-dose" amoxicillin (90 mg/kg/d) became necessary to overcome resistance. The rate of antibiotic-resistant invasive pneumococcal disease has decreased in the post-PCV7 era. However, antibiotic resistance has emerged in serotype 19A. Thus, high-dose amoxicillin dosing is currently the standard of care for suspected bacterial CAP. Amoxicillin/clavulanate, dosed at 90 mg/kg/d for the amoxicillin component, is a reasonable alternative agent.

For children who are initially unable to tolerate oral antibiotics or those with more severe disease, daily therapy with intramuscular ceftriaxone is a viable option in the office setting. In children with hypersensitivity to beta-lactam antibiotics, treatment options include clindamycin, macrolides, fluoroquinolones, and linezolid. However, it should be noted that *S pnuemoniae* resistance to macrolides has remained high and limits the utility of this class of antibiotics in the setting of CAP. For children with more severe disease (complicated by empyema, bacteremia, lung abscess, etc) requiring parenteral therapy, a third-generation cephalosporin (eg, ceftriaxone, cefotaxime) is the drug of choice, often with clindamycin to provide broader coverage including *S aureus* and methicillin-resistant *Staphylococcus aureus* (MRSA). Ampicillin or penicillin G may be used for penicillin-sensitive *S pneumoniae* strains and for children with uncomplicated disease requiring parenteral therapy. Step-down therapy to oral amoxicillin is appropriate for most children in this setting.

Thus, in preschool–aged children with a suspected diagnosis of bacterial CAP, *S pneumoniae* is the most common pathogen and amoxicillin is the empiric antibiotic of choice. Although not all cases of bacterial CAP are caused by *S pneumoniae* and not all isolates will respond to amoxicillin, an appreciation for the clinical presentation and treatment of typical bacterial CAP will allow the clinician to properly treat such cases and recognize the distinguishing features of CAP due to other pathogens.

Suggested Readings

American Academy of Pediatrics. Pneumococcal infections. In: Pickering LK, Baker CJ, Kimberlin DW, Long SS, eds. *Red Book: 2009 Report of the Committee on Infectious Diseases.* 28th ed. Elk Grove Village, IL: American Academy of Pediatrics; 2009:524-535.

Bradley JS, Byington CL, Shah SS, et al. Executive summary: the management of community-acquired pneumonia in infants and children older than 3 months of age: clinical practice guidelines by the pediatric infectious diseases society and the infectious diseases society of America. *Clin Infect Dis.* 2011;53(7):617-630.

Juven T, Mertsola J, Waris M, et al. Etiology of community-acquired pneumonia in 254 hospitalized children. *Pediatr Infect Dis J.* 2000;19(4):293-298.

Kyaw MH, Lynfield R, Schaffner W, et al. Effect of introduction of the pneumococcal conjugate vaccine on drug-resistant *Streptococcus pnuemoniae.* N Engl J Med. 2006;354(14):1455-1463.

Michelow IC, Olsen K, Lozano J, et al. Epidemiology and clinical characteristics of community-acquired pneumonia in hospitalized children. *Pediatrics.* 2004;113(4):701-707.

Whitney CG, Farley MM, Hadler J, et al. Decline in invasive pneumococcal disease after the introduction of protein-polysaccharide conjugate vaccine. *N Engl J Med.* 2003;348(18):1737-1746.

Wubbel L, Muniz L, Ahmed A, et al. Etiology and treatment of community-acquired pneumonia in ambulatory children. *Pediatr Infect Dis J.* 1999;18(2):98-104.

QUESTION 38

When Should Concern Arise About Staphylococcus aureus in a Patient With Pneumonia?

Christopher R. Cannavino, MD

Staphylococcus aureus is an uncommon, but important cause of community-acquired pneumonia (CAP) in children. In recent years, the emergence of community-acquired methicillin-resistant *S aureus* (CA-MRSA) strains in the United States, most of which represent the "USA 300" strain, has heightened the significance of the pathogen in CAP. There are a number of clinical features that are suggestive of *S aureus* infection. Children with *S aureus* pneumonia typically present acutely with rapidly progressive disease. Coinfection with influenza results in particularly severe infection and is associated with significant morbidity and mortality. Given the potential for rapid progression to respiratory failure, a clinical presentation consistent with *S aureus* pneumonia requires prompt recognition and intervention.

S aureus is a catalase-positive, coagulase-positive, gram-positive cocci that forms grape-like clusters. It can asymptomatically colonize the skin and mucous membranes of children. Transmission typically occurs via contact with colonized or infected individuals. Although children with underlying disease (eg, immunosuppression, chronic lung disease) are at higher risk for *S aureus* pneumonia, the majority of cases occur in previously healthy children. Groups at increased risk for infection include young children (particularly infants) and children with prior skin infections. Primary *S aureus* pneumonia can occur after aspiration of the bacteria from the upper respiratory tract or via hematogenous seeding of lungs during periods of bacteremia. Pneumonia may occur in association with an antecedent or concomitant viral infection, particularly influenza. This association with respiratory viral pathogens produces a seasonal peak in *S aureus* pneumonia that mirrors the pattern of viral infections within the community. In children with an influenza-like illness who experience an acute deterioration in their respiratory symptoms, a high index of suspicion for *S aureus* pneumonia should be maintained.

Historically, non-USA 300 MRSA strains were confined to the hospital environment and were most commonly seen in health care–associated infections (eg, ventilator-associated pneumonia). However, in recent years, community-acquired USA 300 MRSA strains have emerged. CA-MRSA was first described in the pediatric population in the 1980s with severe disease and deaths first reported in 1998. Since that time, CA-MRSA has become widespread. Young children (younger than 2 years) have a higher incidence of CA-MRSA disease compared with older children and adults. The majority of the pediatric CA-MRSA disease burden consists of skin-soft tissue infections. However, CA-MRSA has a broad range of potentially severe clinical manifestations associated with significant morbidity and mortality, including severe pneumonia. In the United States, the USA 300 clone of CA-MRSA has virulence factors, including Panton-Valentine leukocidin (PVL), which are likely to be associated with increased pathogenicity. These strains often cause severe, necrotizing pneumonia with bilateral parenchymal disease that frequently results in respiratory failure. Of note, some methicillin-sensitive *S aureus* strains also have PVL genes and may cause indistinguishable clinical infections.

Despite the emergence of CA-MRSA, *S aureus* remains an uncommon cause of CAP. However, *S aureus* pneumonia is associated with significant morbidity and mortality. The typical clinical course of *S aureus* pneumonia is rapidly progressive and severe. Children often present with high fever, cough, and tachypnea, which progresses to significant respiratory distress. Vomiting, abdominal distension, and abdominal pain are variably present. Hypoxemia and complications of pneumonia (eg, parapneumonic effusion, empyema) may emerge over the course of hours. Sepsis and necrotizing pneumonia are common, particularly with CA-MRSA infection. As a result, intensive care unit (ICU) admission and mechanical ventilation are required in many patients with *S aureus* pneumonia. *S aureus* should be suspected in children who present with an acute onset of severe, rapidly progressive signs and symptoms.

When *S aureus* pneumonia is suspected, laboratory and radiographic analysis should be pursued and may prove revealing. Laboratory analysis may reveal profound leukocytosis or leukopenia and markedly increased inflammatory markers (eg, C-reactive protein). Blood cultures are not uncommonly positive, but should be obtained to aid in diagnosis and treatment as a positive blood culture provides a definitive diagnosis and helps guide therapy. Radiographic features include patchy alveolar infiltrates that rapidly progress to form large lobar or multilobar consolidations. Necrotizing pneumonia, or less commonly lung abscess, may be appreciated on computerized tomography imaging. Features of complicated pneumonia are commonly present, including parapneumonic effusions and empyemas. When obtained, pleural fluid cultures are frequently positive. The presence of a pneumatocele is suggestive of *S aureus* pneumonia, and spontaneous pneumothoraces may occur. There has been an increase in *S aureus*, particularly CA-MRSA, complicated pneumonias in recent years. Thus, the presence of a complicated pneumonia should raise suspicion for *S aureus*.

When there is a clinical suspicion for *S aureus* pneumonia, empiric therapy should include antistaphylococcal antibiotics, with consideration for CA-MRSA coverage. Given the potential for rapid deterioration, there should be a low threshold to hospitalize the child for parenteral antibiotics and close monitoring. For severe disease, vancomycin is currently recommended as the preferred treatment for children with MRSA pneumonia. Some experts advocate a combination of a beta-lactamase-resistant beta-lactam antibiotic (eg, nafcillin) and vancomycin or clindamycin (depending on local resistance rates) for empiric intravenous treatment, often in combination with ceftriaxone until the pathogen has been identified. A significant percentage of children with *S aureus* pneumonia require ICU admission, mechanical ventilation, or drainage of parapneumonic effusions (eg, video-assisted thoracoscopic surgery or fibrinolytic therapy with chest tube drainage).

Thus, *S aureus* pneumonia should be considered in children with rapidly progressive or complicated pneumonia, those with known risk factors, or those who do not respond to initial antibiotic therapy. Similarly, *S aureus* should be suspected in children with an influenza-like illness who experience an acute deterioration. CA-MRSA has emerged as an important cause of CAP in recent years and should be taken into consideration when selecting empiric antibiotics in children with severe pneumonia. A high index of suspicion should be maintained in any child with a clinical presentation suggestive of *S aureus* because prompt recognition and intervention is critical.

Suggested Readings

American Academy of Pediatrics. Staphylococcal infections. In: Pickering LK, Baker CJ, Kimberlin DW, et al. eds. *Red Book: 2009 Report of the Committee on Infectious Diseases*. 28th ed. Elk Grove Village, IL: American Academy of Pediatrics; 2009:601-615.

Bradley JS, Byington CL, Shah SS, et al. Executive summary: the management of community-acquired pneumonia in infants and children older than 3 months of age: clinical practice guidelines by the pediatric infectious diseases society and the infectious diseases society of America. *Clin Infect Dis*. 2011;53(7):617-630.

Carrillo-Marquez MA, Hulten KG, Hammerman W, et al. *Staphylococcus aureus* pneumonia in children in the era of community-acquired methicillin-resistance at Texas Children's Hospital. *Pedaitr Infect Dis J*. 2011;30(7): 545-550.

Finelli L, Fiore A, Dhara R, et al. Influenza-associated pediatric mortality in the United States: increase of *Staphylococcus aureus* coinfection. *Pediatrics*. 2008;122(4):805-811.

Gillet Y, Issartel B, Vanhems P, et al. Association between *Staphylococcus aureus* strains carrying GENE for Panton-Valentine leukocidin and highly lethal necrotizing pneumonia in young immunocompetent patients. *Lancet*. 2002;359(9308):753-759.

Herold BC, Immergluck LC, Maranan MC, et al. Community-acquired methicillin-resistant *Staphylococcus aureus* in children with no identified predisposing risk. *JAMA*. 1998;279(8):593-598.

Liu C, Bayer A, Cosgrove SE, et al. Clinical practice guidelines by the Infectious Diseases Society of America for the treatment of methicillin-resistant *Staphylococcus aureus* infections in adults and children: executive summary. *Clin Infect Dis*. 2011;52(3):285-292.

SECTION XII

EPSTEIN-BARR VIRUS/ CYTOMEGALOVIRUS

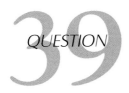

QUESTION

39

WHEN ARE STEROIDS INDICATED IN THE SETTING OF KNOWN ACUTE EPSTEIN-BARR VIRUS INFECTION?

Masako Shimamura, MD and Rebecca W. Widener, MD

Infectious mononucleosis, caused by Epstein-Barr virus, is generally characterized by a triad of pharyngitis, fatigue, and cervical lymphadenopathy. Fever and splenomegaly are also common in presentation. These are symptoms primarily manifested by the host response rather than direct viral infection. The severity and duration of symptoms are variable and most commonly resolve by 2 to 3 months postinfection. However, some (such as lymphadenopathy and fatigue) may persist. Treatment is generally supportive and consists of rest (although strict bed rest is not necessary), over-the-counter symptomatic relief for fever and throat pain, and avoidance of contact sports until the patient is asymptomatic and, if splenomegaly is present, you are no longer able to palpate the spleen.

The use of steroids for treatment of infectious mononucleosis has long been controversial. As early as the 1960s, several studies have sought to provide the answer to this question. A Cochrane review most recently evaluated 7 randomized, controlled trials comparing the effectiveness of corticosteroid regimens to that of placebo. Two of these trials showed no difference between steroid treatment and placebo in regards to the time to resolution of clinical symptoms; one specifically evaluated the use of a combined treatment regimen consisting of acyclovir and prednisolone.[1] Two trials showed initial short-term improvement in sore throat with corticosteroid treatment, although this effect was not sustained. Three trials showed shortened duration in fever with treatment versus placebo; however, the effects on other clinical symptoms such as fatigue and sore throat varied. Overall, as the authors concluded, there were insufficient data throughout these studies to support steroid use in the routine treatment of infectious mononucleosis. The studies were generally small ($n = 24$ to 94) and had variability in the type of corticosteroid used, route of administration, dose, duration, and outcome measures.[2]

The lack of clear evidence of benefit has led to universal recommendations indicating that steroids have no role in the routine use of treatment of infectious mononucleosis.

185

However, despite this, steroids continue to be used somewhat liberally in uncomplicated cases, perhaps to hasten return to school and normal activities because of persistent symptoms, patient demand, or the physician's personal experience, clinical judgment, or training.[3] Steroids are not without adverse effects. Rare case reports have linked the use of steroids for routine mononucleosis with myocarditis, mostly mild and asymptomatic, but causing supraventricular tachycardia in 1 case,[4] and neurologic complications including meningoencephalitis, seizures, and brachial plexus palsy.[5,6] Furthermore, the potential that they may interfere with the immunobiology of the disease has also been theorized, adversely affecting latently infected lymphocytes and long-term immunity.[7] In 1 study of corticosteroid therapy, lymphocytes from young adult patients treated with a 10-day prednisone taper were compared over time to those from untreated patients with severe EBV disease.[8] For the first 2 weeks, lymphocyte totals and subsets were similar between treated and untreated patients, but between weeks 3 and 12 posttreatment, lymphocyte total numbers and subsets of B cells, helper T cells, and cytotoxic T cells were significantly lower in the prednisone-treated group. Although this reduction may contribute to improvement of immune-mediated symptoms, the authors expressed concern regarding the unknown effect of altering the T-lymphocyte response in steroid-treated subjects, as T cells are critical in long-term control of EBV infection in the host. For these reasons, avoidance of routine use of steroids is recommended.

Most patients with an acute EBV infection have a self-limited course and recover without sequelae. Rarely, however, severe complications can occur in both healthy and immunocompromised patients. It is during these times that the use of steroids may, indeed, be warranted. Airway obstruction or impending airway obstruction is due to tonsillar hypertrophy and occurs in approximately 3.5% of patients, but has been reported to occur in as many as 25% of cases.[9] Massive splenomegaly and splenic rupture are the other most commonly feared complications. Although mild splenomegaly is a common finding in acute mononucleosis, found in approximately 50% of patients, serious splenic complications are very rare, occurring in less than 1%. Splenic rupture usually is found to occur during the second and third weeks of illness, at the peak of splenomegaly. Neurologic complications occur in less than 1% of patients. Two of the most common neurologic complications are encephalitis and cranial nerve palsies. Other neurologic complications that have been reported are aseptic meningitis, acute disseminated encephalomyelitis, transverse myelitis, Guillain-Barré syndrome, optic neuritis, and Alice-in-Wonderland syndrome (a perceived distortion of object size).[10] Other life-threatening complications reported include myocarditis, fulminant hepatitis, and liver failure, and hematologic manifestations such as hemolytic anemia, idiopathic thrombocytopenic purpura, and hemophagocytic lymphohistiocytosis. These, and other life-threatening complications, are all indications for use of steroid therapy. Steroids have been used anecdotally and in small case series for these indications, but no rigorous studies have been performed to confirm the benefit of steroid use in these situations. Nevertheless, it is expert opinion that steroids may be useful for these potentially life-threatening complications of EBV infection.

References

1. Tynell E, Aurelius E, Brandell A, et al. Acylcovir and prednisolone treatment of acute infectious mononucleosis; a multicenter, double-blind, placebo-controlled study. *J Infect Dis*. 1996;174(2):324-331.
2. Candy B, Hotopf M. Steroids for symptom control in infectious mononucleosis. *Cochrane Database Syst Rev*. 2006;(3):CD004402. doi: 10.1002/14651858.CD004402.pub.2
3. Thompson SK, Doerr TD, Hengerer AS. Infectious mononucleosis and corticosteroids: management practices and outcomes. *Arch Otolaryngol Head Neck Surg*. 2005;131(5):900-904.
4. Andersson J, Ernberg I. Management of Epstein-Barr virus infections. *Am J Med*. 1988;85(2A):107-115.
5. Berg P, Caris TN, Frenkel EP, Shiver CB. Meningoencephalitis in infectious mononucleosis: report of a case treated with cortisone. *JAMA*. 1956;162(9):885-886.
6. Waldo RT. Neurologic complications of infectious mononucleosis after steroid therapy. *South Med J*. 1981;74(9):1159-1160.
7. Straus SE, Cohen JI, Tosato G, Meier J.. NIH conference. Epstein-Barr virus infections: biology, pathogenesis, and management. *Ann Intern Med*. 1993;118(1):45-58.
8. Brandfonbrener A, Epstein A, Wu S, Phair J. Corticosteroid therapy in Epstein-Barr virus infection. Effect on lymphocyte class, subset, and response to early antigen. *Arch Intern Med*. 1986;146(2):337-339.
9. Wohl DL, Isaacson JE. Airway obstruction in children with infectious mononucleosis. *Ear Nose Throat J*. 1995;74(9):630-638.
10. Doja A, Bitnun A, Ford Jones EL, et al. Pediatric Epstein-Barr virus-associated encephalitis: 10-year review. *J Child Neurol*. 2006:21(5);384-391.

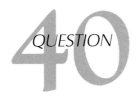
WHAT LABORATORY TEST(S) SHOULD BE OBTAINED IN THE SETTING OF SUSPECTED CONGENITAL CYTOMEGALOVIRUS INFECTION?

Masako Shimamura, MD, and Rebecca W. Widener, MD

Cytomegalovirus (CMV) causes congenital infection in approximately 1% of newborn infants and is a leading cause of neurologic damage and sensorineural hearing loss due to congenital infections.[1] Approximately 10% of neonates born with congenital CMV infection will have symptoms at birth. Symptoms are a result of viral replication and may manifest as intrauterine growth retardation, microcephaly, ventriculomegaly, cerebral calcifications, chorioretinitis, hepatosplenomegaly, jaundice, thrombocytopenia, and petechiae. The remaining 90% of neonates with congenital CMV infection are asymptomatic at birth; however, 5% to 15% of these silent infections will develop neurologic sequelae within several years, primarily sensorineural hearing loss.[2]

If congenital CMV infection is suspected based on maternal exposure or symptoms of the neonate, the gold standard for diagnosis is isolation of the virus from urine or saliva within the first 21 days of life.[3] Infants who are congenitally infected shed large amounts of the virus in the urine and saliva, making both sources easily accessible and detectable. Stool, respiratory secretions, and cerebrospinal fluid (CSF) can also be sent for viral isolation. Traditional cell culture for CMV requires up to 4 weeks for viral detection. For this reason, the shell vial assay is now routinely used for the isolation of CMV virus. Here, tissue culture cells are inoculated with the patient's urine or saliva specimen, centrifuged to enhance viral attachment to the cells, incubated, then stained with anti-CMV monoclonal antibodies. The shell vial assay allows for a diagnosis as early as 24 hours after sample collection.[4] The sensitivity of the assay is quite high, detecting 68% of positive samples within 24 hours and 96% of samples within 48 hours.[5] The culture should be obtained within the first 3 weeks of life in order to confirm the congenital nature of the infection. Outside of the 3-week window of testing, a positive result may be due to either congenital or postnatally acquired infection, and therefore cannot absolutely confirm the diagnosis of congenital CMV. CMV DNA detection in blood, urine, and saliva via polymerase chain reaction (PCR) has also been utilized on a research basis by some investigators; however, this technique has not yet been validated for use in the diagnosis of congenital infection and is not currently recommended to diagnose congenital CMV infection. Serologies are not generally used in infants to diagnose congenital CMV infection. Presence of IgG in the infant could be attributed to maternal transplacentally transmitted antibodies, which could reflect either distant or recent infection and thus cannot be used to determine congenital infection. The commercially available ELISA test for anti-CMV IgM antibodies suffers from both false-positive and false-negative results, rendering interpretation difficult, and therefore is not utilized for diagnosis of congenital CMV infection.[4] Therefore, at this time, culture of the infant's urine or saliva in the first 21 days of life remains the criterion standard for diagnosis of congenital CMV infection.

Further work-up on the infant suspected of having congenital CMV also is recommended. The birth weight, height, and head circumference percentiles should be determined to evaluate for evidence of intrauterine growth retardation. Ancillary tests obtained should also include a complete blood count and liver function tests. If the diagnosis is strongly suspected or confirmed, then a head ultrasound evaluating for ventriculomegaly or parenchymal calcifications and a dilated ophthalmologic examination evaluating retinal involvement should also be performed. The routine newborn hearing screen is, of course, important in the newborn suspected to have congenital CMV. It should be emphasized that in the asymptomatic infant, sensorineural hearing loss can develop in up to 15%, despite normal initial evaluations in the newborn nursery; hearing loss can vary from mild to profound and approximately 50% of infants will develop bilateral hearing loss. Progressive deterioration of hearing loss as well as new, late-onset hearing loss is common over the first years of life. If congenital CMV is confirmed, whether symptomatic or asymptomatic, then serial audiologic evaluations are imperative, especially during the first 3 years of life.[6]

Prenatal testing for congenital CMV infection is controversial. Maternal antibodies drawn during pregnancy can be difficult to interpret. IgM to CMV cannot reliably predict an acute primary infection for the following reasons: (1) in response to a primary infection it can be detected for up to a year, which may precede the time of conception; (2) it can be produced during reactivated, nonprimary infections; and (3) false-positive IgM results can occur from other viral infections such as Parvovirus B19 or Epstein-Barr virus (EBV). Inasmuch as a primary CMV infection would be concerning for transmitting congenital infection to the unborn child, reactivation of prior disease also carries with it a chance of fetal morbidity. Thus, seroimmunity does not confer complete protection from transmitting the virus to the fetus. To help identify primary maternal CMV disease, the CMV IgG avidity test has been used as an adjunctive test on a research basis when the maternal IgM is positive. Initially after primary infection, IgG antibodies exhibit low-avidity binding to CMV antigens; later, refinement of the IgG response favors the production of antibodies with high binding avidity to CMV antigens. Distinction can be made by enzyme immunoassay using a high stringency urea wash to displace low-avidity IgG. Therefore, a low IgG avidity suggests recent, acute disease and a high avidity suggests a nonacute infection. One study has found a 100% sensitivity of the avidity test if used between 16 and 18 weeks gestation; this decreases to a 60% sensitivity after 20 weeks.[7] Avidity testing has been used for research purposes, but it is not widely available on a commercial basis and is not in general use for clinical care purposes. To assess for actual viral transmission to the fetus, an amniocentesis for viral culture and/or PCR may be performed. Testing should be undertaken after 21 weeks gestation (as virus is excreted through fetal urine) and at least 5 to 6 weeks after the proposed maternal infection, when the virus would be present at sufficient quantities in amniotic fluid for detection. Amniocentesis has been shown to have a 100% negative predictive value. It should be emphasized that quantitative viral load in the fetus has not been correlated with symptomatic congenital outcomes. Ultrasound and fetal magnetic resonance imaging (MRI) have been used as anatomical screening tools for positive maternal and/or fetal tests. However, both imaging modalities have poor sensitivity and specificity.[8] Maternal treatment for the possibility of congenital CMV remains controversial and experimental as well. Intravenous immunoglobulin (IVIG) has been used anecdotally in pregnant women thought to be carrying a fetus with congenital CMV infection, but use of IVIG has not been rigorously studied and has no proven benefit. Ganciclovir is contraindicated during pregnancy because it has been assigned to pregnancy category C by the Food Drug Administration (FDA) due to evidence of embryolethality, fetotoxicity, teratogenicity, and mutagenicity in animal models. Currently, the Centers for Disease Control (CDC) does not recommend routine prenatal CMV screening.

References

1. Boppana SB, Pass RF, Britt WJ, Stagno S, Alford CA. Symptomatic congenital cytomegalovirus infection: neonatal morbidity and mortality. *Pediatr Infec Dis J*. 1992;11(2):93-99.
2. Alford CA, Stagno S, Pass RF, Britt WJ. Congenital and perinatal cytomegalovirus infections. *Rev Infect Dis*. 1990;12(7):S745-S753.
3. Best JM. Laboratory diagnosis of congenital and perinatal virus infections. *Clin Diagn Virol*. 1996; 5(2-3):121-129.
4. Demmler GJ. Infectious Diseases Society of America and Centers for Disease Control: summary of a workshop on surveillance for congenital cytomegalovirus disease. *Rev Infect Dis*. 1991;13(2):315-329.
5. Rabella N, Drew WL. Comparison of conventional and shell vial cultures for detecting cytomegalovirus infection. *J Clin Microbiol*. 1990;28(4):806-807.
6. Fowler KB, McCollister FP, Dahle AJ, Boppana S, Britt WJ, Pass RF. Progressive and fluctuating sensorineural hearing loss in children with asymptomatic congenital cytomegalovirus infection. *J Pediatr*. 1997;130(4):624-630.
7. Lazzarotto T, Varani S, Spezzacatena P, et al. Maternal IgG avidity and IgM detected by blot as diagnostic tools to identify pregnant women at risk of transmitting cytomegalovirus. *Viral Immunol*. 2000;13:137-141.
8. Coll O, Benoist G, Ville Y, et al. Recommendations and guidelines for perinatal practice: guidelines on CMV congenital infection. *J Perinat. Med*. 2009;37:433-445.

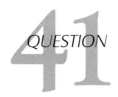

QUESTION

WHEN SHOULD SEROLOGIC TESTING BE PERFORMED INSTEAD OF A MONOSPOT, AND HOW DO I INTERPRET RESULTS OF EPSTEIN-BARR VIRUS SEROLOGIES?

Masako Shimamura, MD and Rebecca W. Widener, MD

Epstein-Barr virus (EBV) is a gamma-herpes virus that establishes a lifelong infection. Transmission usually occurs by the oral route via infected secretions, most commonly saliva. The epidemiology of transmission varies between developing and developed countries. In developing countries, the majority of children become seropositive during early childhood. These transmissions are largely asymptomatic and are thought to occur through infected oral secretions among household contacts. In contrast, in developed countries transmission is delayed such that only about half of the population is seropositive by adolescence. Primary EBV infection during adolescence is more often symptomatic compared to that acquired in early childhood, resulting in symptoms and signs of infectious mononucleosis (IM). These may include headache, malaise, fatigue, fever, sore throat, lymphadenopathy, jaundice, rash, hepatosplenomegaly, and eyelid edema.

EBV infects B lymphocytes via the CD21 receptor, initially in the tonsillar epithelium and later in peripheral circulation. There is a 4- to 6-week incubation period between primary inoculation and clinical symptoms of IM. Like other herpes viruses, EBV gene transcripts are categorized by temporal kinetics into immediate-early, early, and late genes, with full expression occurring during lytic infection resulting in production of infectious virions. Immediate-early and early gene products activate viral and cellular gene transcription and modify the cellular environment for viral persistence and replication. Late gene products encode structural virion components including the viral nucleocapsid enclosing the viral DNA, the tegument proteins surrounding the nucleocapsid, and the surface glycoproteins.

Infectious virus can be recovered from oral secretions during IM, but viral culture is rarely performed clinically due to technically demanding aspects of EBV culture in vitro. Infectious virions may also continue to be recoverable intermittently from oral secretions long after IM symptoms subside. EBV immortalizes B cells and latent virus may be

193

detectable by polymerase chain reaction (PCR) in peripheral blood B cells for the life of the host. In latency, only a limited number of viral genes may be transcribed in circulating B cells without production of infectious virions.

During acute IM, EBV stimulates polyclonal activation of B lymphocytes, resulting in a general elevation of IgM, IgG, and IgA. As part of this nonspecific antibody production, heterophile antibodies are produced. Simply stated, heterophile antibodies are those that cross-react to antigens over species lines. More specifically in EBV infection, the heterophile antibody is primarily an IgM antibody that is made in response to an EBV viral surface antigen and has the ability to cross-react with epitopes on nonhuman erythrocytes. The Monospot test is a rapid diagnostic test for EBV IM. It relies on the ability to detect heterophile antibodies in the infected patient's serum. In the case of the Monospot, a latex agglutination test, the nonhuman erythrocytes are equine derived and a positive test yields agglutination of the patient's sera with the equine erythrocyte substrate.

Under appropriate circumstances, heterophile antibody tests are highly sensitive and specific, up to 92% and 100%, respectively.[1] In adolescents and adults, the Monospot has been shown to have a sensitivity of 86% and specificity of 90%. The sensitivity, however, greatly decreases in children younger than 12 years old, to that of 38% (25% to 50% sensitivity range for all the heterophile antibody assays tested).[2] One study evaluating heterophile antibody testing in 44 children younger than 4 years found a sensitivity of 19% to 32%; children older than 4 had sensitivity closer to that of adolescents and adults, at 80% to 84%.[3] In addition to the sensitivity lacking in children, it is also found to be low in adolescents and adults during the first week of illness, with a 25% false-negative rate. This decreases to a 5% to 10% false-negative response by the second week and 5% by the third week of illness.[4] Heterophile antibodies are present during the first month of illness, and then rapidly fall after the fourth week, although they may be detectable in some patients for up to 1 year postinfection. A diagnosis of acute IM can be considered when greater than 10% atypical lymphocytes and a positive heterophile antibody test are observed, regardless of the patient's age.

Some patients with primary EBV infections, particularly young children as discussed above, do not develop heterophile antibodies. Therefore, if the initial heterophile antibody test is negative and your clinical suspicion for primary EBV infection remains, then a set of EBV serologies can be obtained. In addition to EBV serologies, you should also consider evaluating your patients for other causes of heterophile-negative IM, such as cytomegalovirus, toxoplasmosis, HIV, viral hepatitis, adenovirus, and rubella. For EBV, serologic studies consist of 4 antibodies: IgM and IgG to the viral capsid antigen (VCA), IgG to the early antigen (EA), and IgG to EBV nuclear antigen (EBNA) (Table 41-1). IgM VCA arises acutely, then disappears by the fourth to sixth week after onset of symptoms. IgG VCA also appears acutely and peaks by weeks 2 to 4. It will persist for life. IgG EA is seen also during the acute phase and then disappears by 3 to 6 months, although in 20% of people it can persist for years. EBNA antibody is not an acute phase antibody, but appears at 2 to 4 months after onset and persists for life.[5] The antigens against which each of these EBV antibodies reacts are in fact a mixture of related antigenic viral proteins. Thus, the VCA comprises several nucleocapsid proteins (including BcLF1, BFRF3, BLRF2, gp110), which are expressed in lytically infected cells. The EA refers to several immediate-early and early viral proteins (including BZLF1, ABLF2, BHRF1, BMRF1, BMLF1). Similarly, EBNA

Table 41-1
Anti-Epstein-Barr Virus Antibodies During Infectious Mononucleosis

	VCA IgM	*VCA IgG*	*EA IgG*	*EBNA IgG*
Acute infection	+	+	+/−	−
Recent infection	+/−	+	+/−	−
Past infection	−	+	+/−	+
No infection	−	−	−	−

refers to 6 distinct nuclear proteins (EBNA1, 2, 3A, 3B, 3C, -LP), although the reactivity detected by the anti-EBNA assay is largely associated with EBNA1. IgGs directed against VCA and EBNA persist for life, consistent with lifelong persistence of this herpes virus in the healthy host. Some patients may also continue to have positive EA IgG. Therefore, repeated serologic testing of patients after acute EBV IM is not necessary or useful.

The significance of anti-EBV antibodies in long-term control of persistent infection remains unclear, as T lymphocytes are thought to maintain long-term control of EBV in the healthy host. Interestingly, although EBV infects B cells, the atypical lymphocytosis observed during acute IM consists not of B lymphocytes but an expansion of CD8+ cytotoxic T lymphocytes (CTLs). Clinical IM symptoms are induced by cytokines produced by EBV-specific CTLs, rather than direct viral replication. After acute IM, EBV specific memory T cells develop and are thought to maintain long-term control of the virus in the healthy host. Dysregulation of T lymphocytes, as in some primary immundeficiencies (x-linked lymphoproliferative syndrome), after solid organ or stem cell transplantation, or AIDS, is associated with EBV disease and lymphoproliferative syndromes.

References

1. Elgh F, Linderholm M. Evaluation of 6 commercially available kits using purified heterophile antigen for the rapid diagnosis of infectious mononucleosis compared with EBV specific serology. *Clin Diagn Virol.* 1996;7(1):17-21.
2. Linderholm M, Boman J, Juto P, Linde A. Comparative evaluation of nine kits for rapid diagnosis of infectious mononucleosis and Epstein Barr virus-specific serology. *J Clin Microbiol.* 1994;32(1):259-261.
3. Sumaya CV, Ench Y. Epstein-Barr virus infectious mononucleosis in children: II. Heterophil antibody and viral-specific responses. *Pediatrics.* 1985;75(6):1011-1019.
4. Hoagland RJ. Infectious mononucleosis. *Primary Care.* 1975;2(2);295-307.
5. Epstein-Barr virus and Infectious Mononucleosis. Atlanta, GA: Centers for Disease Control and Prevention, National Center for Infectious Diseases. Updated May 16, 2006. http://www.cdc.gov/ncidod/diseases/ebv.htm

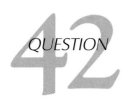
What Should I Tell a Pregnant Mother of a 2 Year Old Who Has Recently Been Diagnosed With Congenital Cytomegalovirus Infection About Her Risk for Developing Infection as Well as Prevention Techniques?

Masako Shimamura, MD and Rebecca W. Widener, MD

In immunocompetent children and adults, including pregnant women, primary congenital cytomegalovirus (CMV) infections most often are asymptomatic. When symptoms do arise, they can manifest nonspecifically as a fever, headache, flu-like illness, or as a heterophile-negative mononucleosis syndrome. Following the primary infection, as with other herpes viruses, CMV establishes lifelong persistent infection characterized by latency interspersed with periodic reactivations. Asymptomatic shedding in the urine and saliva can persist for months in adults and years in children after primary infection. Viral shedding can also occur intermittently with reactivations, which are usually asymptomatic. Due to this asymptomatic shedding, exposure to CMV may occur at any time by contact with infected secretions.

If a pregnant mother is exposed to someone with a known CMV infection, it is important to counsel her on the prevalence of CMV, risk of developing a primary infection, transmission of the virus to the fetus, and preventive strategies to reduce these risks.

Overall, the US seroprevalence to CMV in people age 6 years and older is very common, estimated at 60%[1]; seroimmunity to CMV in pregnant women ranges from 40% to 80%. In women who are seronegative, 2% to 4% will develop a primary CMV infection during pregnancy.[2] Among the general population, seroconversion rates among health care workers are similar to pregnant women, as are the rates for parents who have children not actively shedding CMV. Day care workers have a higher risk of seroconversion with an average annual conversion rate of 8.5%. Risk factors for seroconversion include

---

Table 42-1

Centers for Disease Control Recommendations for Avoidance of Cytomegalovirus-Containing Secretions by Pregnant Women

- Wash hands frequently with soap and water for 15 to 20 seconds, especially after the following:
  - Changing diapers
  - Feeding a young child
  - Wiping a young child's nasal secretions or saliva
  - Handling children's toys
- Avoid sharing food, drinks, or eating utensils used by young children
- Avoid placing a child's pacifier into own mouth
- Avoid sharing toothbrushes with young children
- Avoid contact with saliva when·kissing a young child (includes mouth kissing)
- Clean toys and surfaces that come into contact with children's urine or saliva

Adapted from The Centers for Disease Control and Prevention. *Cytomegalovirus (CMV) and Congenital CMV Infection.* www.cdc.gov/cmv/prevention.html.

---

demographics such as ethnicity and socioeconomic status, sexual activity, and most importantly, having a child in the home who is actively shedding the virus. Group day care attendance is a risk factor for acquisition of CMV among young children, who then may transmit CMV to their seronegative parents. Being a seronegative parent of a child who is actively shedding CMV carries a seroconversion rate of about 25%.[3]

Congenital CMV infections occur through both maternal primary infections and nonprimary infections, which may result from reactivation of a latent virus or with reinfection from a new strain.[4] In developing countries where the seroprevalence among adults approaches 100%, congenital CMV infection still occurs. Thus, maternal immunity prior to conception does not confer complete protection to the fetus from congenital CMV infection. Maternal immune status should be considered when counseling on the rate of transmitting the virus to the unborn child. The intrauterine transmission rate during maternal nonprimary infection is approximately 1%.[5] In contrast, primary CMV infection during pregnancy carries a risk of intrauterine transmission of 30% to 40%. Gestational age has been shown not to be a factor in the rate of transmission; however, when transmission occurs during the first half of pregnancy, symptoms of congenital CMV infection tend to be more severe.[2] It should be noted that unless the pregnant mother was proven to be CMV seronegative just prior to conception and seroconverts during pregnancy, CMV serology drawn during pregnancy is difficult to interpret and is not routinely recommended (see Question 40).

Prevention following exposure to a known infection source focuses on avoidance of contact with urine, feces, and saliva, which may carry infectious virions. These include proper hand hygiene, especially hand washing following diaper changes (Table 42-1). CMV is an enveloped virus, and simple detergents such as household soap can disrupt the viral envelope, rendering the particles noninfectious. Thus, although other viracidal agents such as bleach, chlorhexidine, and alcohol sanitizers are also effective decontaminants, simple hand washing with soap and water is sufficient to remove CMV from the hands after contact with infectious secretions. In addition to decontamination, avoidance of exposure to infected secretions is also advised. Thus, the mother should also be counseled to avoid direct contact with saliva, such as kissing on the mouth or drinking, eating, or sharing utensils after her child. These strategies have been shown to reduce the risk of developing a primary CMV infection in an otherwise seronegative pregnant mother.[6] Because asymptomatic shedding of the virus is so common, no other special precautions are needed during times of primary infection or reactivation, and in fact these avoidance and decontamination measures may be recommended for pregnant women in general due to potential ongoing exposure to unknown CMV-shedding contacts. The same preventive approach is also recommended routinely for pregnant mothers who work in day care centers and hospital environments. Maternal treatment for presumed or proven congenital CMV infection in the fetus has been attempted anecdotally, including use of passive immunoglobulin. No large-scale studies to date have proven substantial benefit, and currently there are no recommendations regarding intrauterine treatment of fetuses with congenital CMV infection. Vaccine studies are also underway, although the progress in this field has been slow, particularly given that maternal natural immunity to CMV does not confer complete protection from intrauterine infection.

Most women have no knowledge of CMV infection, despite it being the most common viral congenital infection and affecting as many infants as Down syndrome or neural tube defects. Both the Centers for Disease Control and Prevention (CDC) and the American College of Obstetrics and Gynecology (ACOG) recommend that obstetricians and gynecologists (OB/GYN) counsel their patients on the prevalence and prevention of CMV. A survey was undertaken in 2007 by the ACOG to assess OB/GYN knowledge of congenital CMV and their practices of counseling on prevention. The survey revealed large gaps in the comprehensive knowledge of CMV modes of transmission and preventive strategies. It also showed that fewer than half of the physicians (44%) counseled their patients on CMV prevention, identifying a need for further training of OB/GYNs in the area of congenital CMV prevention.[7] It should be emphasized, however, that family physicians who practice obstetrics and pediatricians who routinely see the siblings of pregnant mothers should also expand their knowledge on congenital CMV and undertake the important role of counseling their patients on prevention as well.

References

1. Staras SA, Dollard SC, Radford KW, Flanders D, Pass RF, Cannon MJ. Seroprevalence of cytomegalovirus infection in the United States, 1988-1994. *Clin Infect Dis*. 2006;43(9):1143-1151.
2. Stagno S, Pass RF, Cloud G, et al. Primary cytomegalovirus infection in pregnancy: incidence, transmission to fetus, and clinical outcome. *JAMA*. 1986;256(14):1904-1908.

3. Hyde TB, Schmid DS, Cannon MJ. Cytomegalovirus seroconversion rates and risk factors: implication for congenital CMV. *Rev Med Virol.* 2010;20(5):311-326.
4. Boppana S, Rivera LB, Fowler KB, Mach M, Britt WJ. Intrauterine transmission of cytomegalovirus to infants of women with preconceptual immunity. *N Engl J Med.* 2001;344(18):1366-1371.
5. Kenneson A, Cannon MJ. Review and meta-analysis of the epidemiology of congenital cytomegalovirus (CMV) infection. *Rev Med Virol.* 2007;17(4):253-276.
6. Adler SP, Finney JW, Manganello A, Best AM. Prevention of child-to-mother transmission of cytomegalovirus among pregnant women. *J Pediatr.* 2004;145(4):485-491.
7. Centers for Disease Control and Prevention (CDC). Knowledge and practices of obstetricians and gynecologists regarding cytomegalovirus infection during pregnancy—United States, 2007. *MMWR Morb Mortal Wkly Rep.* 2008;57(3):65-68.

SECTION XIII

LYMPHADENOPATHY

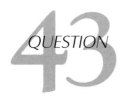
A 13-Year-Old Female Presents With Symptoms of Cat Scratch Disease. What Is the Best Approach to the Diagnosis and the Preferred Management of a Patient With Cat Scratch Disease?

Ankhi Dutta, MD, MPH and Debra L. Palazzi, MD

Cat scratch disease (CSD) is caused by fastidious gram-negative bacilli *Bartonella henselae* and *Bartonella quintana*. Cats are natural reservoirs of *B henselae* with a seroprevalence of 81% in stray cats and 28% in domestic cats in the United States. CSD can occur from a cat scratch or bite, but also may occur from cat flea (*Ctenocephalides felis*) bites.

The diagnosis of CSD should be based on clinical examination findings in addition to laboratory tests. Serology confers the highest yield in the otherwise healthy child with clinical features compatible with infection. The 2 commonly used methods for detecting CSD antibodies are the indirect immunofluorescent antibody test and the enzyme immunoassay. In general, immunoglobulin (Ig)M and IgG antibodies are detectable between 1 and 2 weeks after the onset of symptoms, although IgM antibodies can be undetectable at the time of clinical diagnosis. A *Bartonella* IgG antibody titer more than 1:256 is indicative of an acute infection. Titers between 1:64 and 1:256 suggest possible CSD, and repeat testing is recommended in 10 to 14 days. A titer less than 1:64 generally means absence of infection. The *Bartonella* IgM antibody response is brief, but its presence strongly suggests an acute infection; however, some individuals remain seronegative throughout the entire course of illness.

Serological testing is available through the Centers for Disease Control and Prevention (CDC), State Health Laboratories, as well as many commercial laboratories. However, the testing turnaround time at the CDC generally is longer, requiring 2 to 3 weeks for results. Results may be able to be expedited by calling either your state health laboratory or the CDC.

Figure 43-1. Cat-Scratch Disease (Bartonella henslae) Stellate microabscess and silver-stained coccobacillary forms of Bartonella henselae within the inflammatory infiltrate of the involved lymph node(a, hematoxylin and eosin, original magnification x 12.5). (Reprinted with permission of the American Academy of Pediatrics. Red Book Online Visual Library. Available at: http://aapredbook.aappublications.org/visual.)

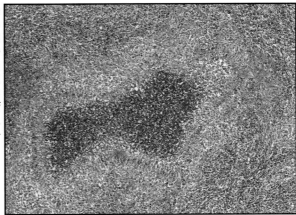

Blood and tissue cultures are unreliable in detecting *Bartonella* species because the organisms are difficult to grow in culture media and require special plating and incubation techniques. Therefore, this method is generally not recommended for diagnosis. Biopsy of an enlarged lymph node or the primary inoculation site may be required for a definitive diagnosis in some patients, particularly those who do not respond to antimicrobial therapy, who have an atypical presentation of disease, or for whom the diagnosis is unclear. Histopathologic examination of a tissue specimen will reveal nonspecific lymphoid hyperplasia in the initial phase of disease followed by noncaseating epithelioid granulomas later in the course of illness (Figure 43-1). Histopathology of the primary inoculation site will show acellular areas of necrosis in the dermis, with histiocytes and epithelioid cells surrounding the areas of necrosis; multinucleated giant cells may or may not be present. Both of the above findings are suggestive of CSD but are nonspecific. Special staining techniques like the Warthin-Starry stain may reveal dark brown to black pleomorphic bacilli in chains, clumps, or filaments but are also nonspecific for CSD.

Recently, polymerase chain reaction (PCR) assays have become available at commercial laboratories and at the CDC. They are highly sensitive and specific for *Bartonella* species, especially when used on tissue specimens and are recommended if tissue is available. A PCR assay on blood specimens also is available through the CDC and commercial laboratories but there are reports of low sensitivity (<20%) in patients with CSD lymphadenitis, and data on clinical utility are limited.

Approximately 25% of patients with *Bartonella* species infection develop complicated disease (Table 43-1). In patients with prolonged fever, abdominal pain, or organomegaly; ultrasound or computed tomography of the abdomen may reveal microabscesses in the liver and spleen (Figure 43-2). This finding, along with the appropriate clinical presentation, may lend additional support to your diagnosis of CSD.

Localized CSD usually is a self-limiting illness with symptoms that resolve spontaneously in 2 to 4 months. Some experts recommend symptomatic treatment of localized CSD adenitis (eg, needle aspiration of suppurated lymph nodes). Although treatment of localized CSD in mildly affected patients is of unproven benefit, some experts recommend treatment of acutely ill patients or those with painfully suppurative lymph nodes with azithromycin (in patients weighing less than 100 lbs: 10 mg/kg PO on day 1, then

Table 43-1

Complicated and Uncomplicated Disease Processes in Cat Scratch Disease, Along With Commonly Used Medications for Treatment

Clinical Disease	Treatment	Route	Duration of Therapy
Lymphadenitis	Azithromycin	PO	5 days
	Alternatives: Clarithromycin **OR** Rifampin **OR** Trimethoprim- sulfamethoxazole **OR** Ciprofloxacin	PO	7 to 10 days
*Hepatosplenic CSD or prolonged fever	Rifampin **PLUS** gentamicin	PO IV	10 to 14 days
	OR		
	Rifampin **PLUS** azithromycin	PO PO	10 to 14 days
*Neuroretinitis	Children <8 years		
	Rifampin **PLUS** azithromycin **OR** trimethoprim- sulfamethoxazole	PO PO	4 to 6 weeks
	Children ≥8 years	PO	4 to 6 weeks
	Doxycycline **PLUS** rifampin	 PO	
*Neurologic disease	Children <8 years		
	Rifampin **PLUS** azithromycin **OR** Trimethoprim-sulfamethoxazole	PO PO	10 to 14 days
	Children ≥8 years		
	Doxycycline **PLUS** rifampin	PO PO	10 to 14 days

(continued)

Table 43-1 (continued)

Complicated and Uncomplicated Disease Processes in Cat Scratch Disease, Along With Commonly Used Medications for Treatment

Clinical Disease	Treatment	Route	Duration of Therapy
*Suspected endocarditis	Ceftriaxone	IV	6 weeks
	PLUS		
	Gentamicin	IV	14 days
	WITH OR WITHOUT		
	Doxycycline	PO	6 weeks (some recommended 3 to 6 months)
*Proven endocarditis	Gentamicin	IV	14 days
	PLUS		
	Doxycycline	PO	
	If cannot receive gentamicin, may use rifampin		6 weeks (some recommended 3 to 6 months)

CSD = cat scratch disease

*Consultation with an infectious diseases specialist is suggested.

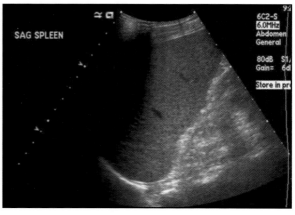

Figure 43-2. Ultrasound of the spleen showing numerous microabscesses. (Reprinted with permission of Ankhi Dutta, MD and Morven Edwards, MD.)

5 mg/kg PO on days 2 to 5; in patients weighing >100 lbs: 500 mg PO on day 1, then 250 mg PO on days 2 to 5) or trimethoprim-sulfamethoxazole (trimethoprim component 8 mg/kg/d in 2 divided doses for 7 to 10 days). Commonly used alternative antibiotics for treating CSD include rifampin, ciprofloxacin, doxycycline, and clarithromycin. Beta-lactam antibiotics, despite in vitro susceptibility testing that is favorable, are ineffective in treating CSD. The optimal drug and duration of treatment is unknown. Incision and drainage of lymph nodes should be avoided due to the risk of forming draining sinuses and fistulas.

Antimicrobial therapy is recommended in patients with systemic symptoms, painful adenopathy, hepatosplenic CSD, all immunocompromised patients and patients with complicated CSD. Little is known about the optimal therapy and duration of treatment. Patients with complicated CSD including those with hepatosplenic involvement, endocarditis, neurologic symptoms, or neuroretinitis should be referred to an infectious disease specialist for evaluation and appropriate treatment, which generally requires combination antimicrobial therapy for 2 to 6 weeks depending on the organ involvement and clinical course. Table 43-1 describes the treatment options available for children with localized as well as systemic CSD.

Suggested Readings

Agan BK, Dolan MJ. Laboratory diagnosis of *Bartonella* infections. *Clin Lab Med.* 2002;22(4):937-962.

American Academy of Pediatrics. Cat scratch disease (Bartonella henselae). In: Pickering LK, ed. *2009 Red Book: Report of the Committee on Infectious Diseases.* 28th Ed. Elk Grove Village, Ill: American Academy of Pediatrics; 2009:249-250.

Bass JW, Freitas BC, Freitas AD. Prospective randomized double-blind placebo-controlled evaluation of azithromycin for treatment of cat-scratch disease. *Pediatr Infect Dis J.* 1998;17(6):447-452.

Margileth AM. Antibiotic therapy for cat scratch disease: clinical study of therapeutic outcome in 268 patients and a review of the literature. *Pediatr Infect Dis J.* 1992;11(6):474-478.

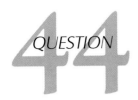
WHAT ARE THE MOST COMMON PATHOGENS AND EMPIRIC TREATMENT(S) OF CHOICE IN A PATIENT WITH SUSPECTED ACUTE BACTERIAL LYMPHADENITIS?

Ankhi Dutta, MD, MPH and Debra L. Palazzi, MD

Lymphadenitis is defined as a tender, enlarged, and inflamed lymph node. It is important to elicit a complete history and physical examination in a child with lymphadenitis. In order to formulate a differential diagnosis of lymphadenitis, the following clinical features should be considered: (1) the patient's age; (2) the size, location, and consistency of the lymph node; (3) whether it is generalized or localized, unilateral or bilateral; (4) the duration of enlargement or inflammation; (5) the associated symptoms; and (6) the social history, including pets, travel, and immunization status. The differential diagnosis of lymphadenopathy is broad. Noninfectious causes include malignancies and immunologic disorders. Infection of lymph nodes can be caused by bacteria, viruses, fungi, and parasites. The bacterial causes of acute lymphadenitis in children are as follows:

- *Staphylococcus aureus* **and Group A** *Streptococcus* **(GAS)**: These 2 pathogens account for the majority (up to 80%) of acute bacterial lymphadenitis in children. Submandibular lymph nodes are the most commonly affected. The involved node is erythematous, warm, and tender to touch and may become fluctuant over time. Patients may present with severe torticollis caused by suppuration of the lymph nodes and surrounding inflammation. Associated symptoms can include fever, recent upper respiratory tract illness, or impetigo. Physical examination may reveal acute otitis media, pharyngitis, or tonsillitis in addition to lymph node swelling, tenderness, and erythema. Lymphadenopathy is most commonly unilateral.
- **Group B** *Streptococcus* **(GBS)**: GBS-associated lymphadenitis occurs in infants, most commonly between the ages of 2 to 3 weeks. Typically, the infant has an acute onset of fever, poor feeding, and irritability with unilateral lymphadenitis. Most commonly there is facial and submandibular cellulitis (cellulitis-adenitis syndrome) with or without ipsilateral otitis media. Patients can be bacteremic (80% to 90%) and have associated meningitis (25%).

- **Anaerobes:** Anaerobic bacteria (*Peptostreptococcus*, *Propionibacteria*, *Bacteroides*, *Fusobacteria*) are important pathogens causing unilateral cervical lymphadenitis in the setting of dental or periondontal infections in older children. A thorough examination of the oral cavity in patients with unilateral cervical adenitis to look for dental caries or periodontal abscesses should be performed. If untreated, these infections can have serious consequences, including jugular vein thrombophlebitis with or without septic pulmonary emboli (Lemierre syndrome) or extension into the central nervous system or mediastinum. Most often these infections are polymicrobial, and associated bacteremia may be present.
- *Yersinia pestis:* Bubonic plague is the most common form of infection caused by *Y pestis*. It usually manifests as an exquisitely tender, nonfluctuant, nonsuppurative lymphadenitis (bubo) involving the regional lymph nodes, following a flea (from wild mammals, cats, and dogs) bite. A detailed social history is important, and travel to the southwestern United States or a history of skinning and handling wild animals in a patient with consistent physical examination findings is suggestive of bubonic plague. Most often the bubo is unilateral. Associated symptoms include high fever, chills, headache, malaise, and vomiting. Immediate hospitalization is indicated because bubonic plague can rapidly progress to shock and death.
- *Francisella tularensis:* Ulceroglandular and glandular forms of tularemia are the most common manifestations. Important clues to the diagnosis include a history of a tick bite, exposure to rabbits or squirrels, or consumption of raw or undercooked game meat. Children usually present with multiple enlarged and tender lymph nodes usually in the inguinal, cervical, or axillary regions. Associated symptoms include fever, chills, malaise, and gastrointestinal symptoms. On physical examination, intact or ulcerated papules with raised edges may be found distal to involved lymph nodes. In the oculoglandular form of tularemia, nodules and ulcers are present on the conjuctiva along with tender preauricular lymphadenitis.

Subacute or chronic causes of bacterial adenitis include *Bartonella* species, nontuberculous mycobacteria, and *Mycobacterium tuberculosis*. Other uncommon causes of bacterial lymphadenitis include actinomycoses, *Nocardia*, occasionally brucellosis, *Yersinia* enterocolitica, other gram-negative bacilli, *Listeria monocytogenes*, other streptococci, and rarely *Staphylococcus epidermidis*.

Treatment

When a child presents with an acute onset of localized lymphadenitis, empiric therapy with an antimicrobial agent that treats the most common causative organisms such as GAS and *Staphylococcus aureus* is a reasonable approach. Clindamycin and trimethoprim-sulfamethoxazole are good options with the increase in prevalence of methicillin-resistant *S aureus* (MRSA) across the United States. However, it is important to remember that trimethoprim-sulfamethoxazole does not treat GAS infection. In regions with a low prevalence of MRSA, a first-generation cephalosporin can be used and will cover both methicillin-susceptible *S aureus* and GAS. A throat swab for a rapid streptococcal antigen

Table 44-1
Treatment Guidelines for Acute Bacterial Adenitis

Pathogen	Clinical Status	Empirical Therapy
SA or GAS	Nontoxic, minimal to moderate cellulitis	Oral clindamycin or TMP-SMX (SA only) or cephalexin (except for MRSA)
	Moderate-severe cellulitis, suppuration	Incision/drainage, IV clindamycin, oxacillin, nafcillin, or vancomycin
GBS	Infants with facial or neck cellulitis with or without systemic symptoms	IV penicillin or ampicillin
Anaerobes	Dental or periodontal disease, nontoxic Toxic, other complications like Lemierre syndrome (concern for polymicrobial infections)	Oral clindamycin or penicillin with β-lactamase inhibitor (amoxicillin-clavulanate) IV vancomycin **AND** IV penicillin with β-lactamase inhibitor (piperacillin-tazobactam or ticarcillin-clavulanate) **OR** metronidazole + a third generation cephalosporin (ceftriaxone or cefotaxime)
Tularemia	Treat in all cases	IV streptomycin Alternatives: IV gentamicin, ciprofloxacin, tetracyclines, or chloramphenicol
Yersinia pestis	Treat in all cases	IV gentamicin or doxycycline Alternatives: TMP-SMX or chloramphenicol

SA: *Staphylococcus aureus*; GAS: Group A *Streptococcus*; MRSA: Methicillin-resistant *Staphylococcus aureus*; GBS: Group B *Streptococcus*; TMP-SMX: trimethoprim-sulfamethoxazole

test and throat culture can be obtained to look for evidence of GAS. If GAS is found to be the causative organism, penicillin remains a first-line therapy because resistance has never been documented (Table 44-1).

Clinical improvement should be monitored for 48 to 72 hours. If the node becomes fluctuant, incision and drainage should be performed and purulent material sent for culture.

However, if the clinical presentation is subacute or chronic and suspicion of *Bartonella* species or nontuberculous mycobacteria is high, this procedure should be avoided to prevent fistula or sinus tract formation. Excisional biopsy is the treatment of choice in the setting of nontuberculous mycobacteria infection.

If response to oral antibiotic therapy is noted, continuation for a total of 10 days is typically sufficient. If response to antibiotic therapy is not seen or the clinical status worsens, treatment with intravenous vancomycin or a semisynthetic penicillin (oxacillin or nafcillin) may be warranted. A complete blood count and a blood culture should be obtained in hospitalized patients with systemic symptoms. Ultrasound or computed tomography of the lymph node(s) can be performed to evaluate for a drainable fluid collection, and surgical consultation requested for significant findings.

Lymphadenitis caused by anaerobic bacteria should be treated empirically with clindamycin or amoxicillin-clavulanate. If the node(s) is fluctuant, needle aspiration or incision and drainage when applicable should be performed and purulent material sent for anaerobic as well as routine cultures. Once the organisms are identified and antimicrobial susceptibilities are known, penicillin may be an option for therapy.

Suggested Readings

Friedmann AM. Evaluation and management of lymphadenopathy in children. *Pediatr Rev.* 2008;29(2):53-60.

Healy CM, Baker CJ. Cervical adenitis. In: Feigin RD, Cherry JD, Demmler-Harrison GJ, Kaplan SL, eds. *Textbook of Pediatric Infectious Diseases.* 6th ed. PA: Elsevier Saunders; 2009:185-197.

Thorell EA, Chesney PJ. Cervical lymphadenitis and neck infections. In: Long SS, Pickering LK, Prober CG, eds. *Principles and Practice of Pediatric Infectious Diseases.* JFK Boulevard, PA: Churchill Livingstone Elsevier Science; 2008:143-155.

SECTION XIV

PROLONGED FEVER

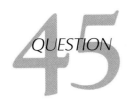

WHAT IS THE DIFFERENTIAL DIAGNOSIS IN A 3-YEAR-OLD FEMALE WITH A 7-DAY HISTORY OF FEVER, RED EYES AND LIPS, RASH, AND SWOLLEN HANDS?

Laura Patricia Stadler, MEd, MD, MS

In this clinical setting, it is most prudent to rule out the possibility of Kawasaki disease (KD), as it is the leading cause of acquired cardiac disease in children in the United States. KD was first described in 1969 by Dr. Tomisaku Kawasaki as a lymphomucocutaneous syndrome in which individuals have fever, an irritable or toxic clinical presentation, and supporting symptoms. The diagnosis of KD has largely been based on the presence of fever for 5 days and 4 of 5 classically described symptoms:

1. Bilateral injection of the conjunctivae, which is characteristically nonexudative and *spares* the limbus (Figure 45-1).
2. Mucous membrane changes including erythema, swelling, and/or cracked lips, "strawberry tongue" without oral ulcers or exudative pharyngitis (Figure 45-1).
3. Maculopapular rash, which may have perineal involvement and/or enhancement (Figure 45-2).
4. Extremity changes including impressive edema and/or erythema of hands and feet (Figure 45-3) as well as periungual desquamation (more often seen ~week 2 of illness) (Figure 45-4).
5. Cervical lymph node ≥1.5 cm, usually unilateral.

Given that a child may not manifest 4 of the 5 symptoms simultaneously, a definitive cause (and thus diagnostic testing) has not been determined, and the significant morbidity and mortality if KD is undetected, the American Heart Association (AHA) developed an algorithm in 2004 to help guide health care professionals with the evaluation of suspected incomplete KD (Figure 45-5). This algorithm provides a guide of supplemental laboratory tests and diagnostics such as an echocardiogram that may be supportive of a diagnosis of incomplete KD.

215

Figure 45-1. Clinical manifestations of Kawasaki disease: Conjunctival injection, lip edema, and erythema in a 2-year-old boy on the sixth day of illness. (Reprinted with permission of the Council on Cardiovascular Disease in the Young, Committee on Rheumatic Fever, Endocarditis, and Kawasaki Disease, American Heart Association Diagnostic Guidelines for Kawasaki Disease. *Circulation.* 2001;103:335-336.)

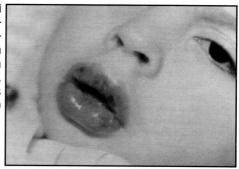

Figure 45-2. Clinical manifestations of Kawasaki disease: Rash of Kawasaki disease in a 7-month-old on the fourth day of illness. (Reprinted with permission of the Council on Cardiovascular Disease in the Young, Committee on Rheumatic Fever, Endocarditis, and Kawasaki Disease, American Heart Association Diagnostic Guidelines for Kawasaki Disease. *Circulation.* 2001;103:335-336.)

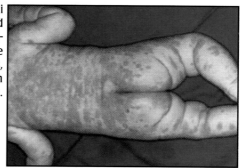

Figure 45-3. Clinical manifestations of Kawasaki disease: Erythematous and edematous hand of a 1.5-year-old girl on the sixth day of illness. (Reprinted with permission of the Council on Cardiovascular Disease in the Young, Committee on Rheumatic Fever, Endocarditis, and Kawasaki Disease, American Heart Association Diagnostic Guidelines for Kawasaki Disease. *Circulation.* 2001;103:335-336.)

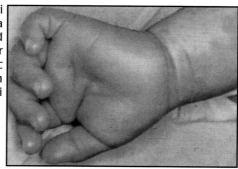

Figure 45-4. Clinical manifestations of Kawasaki disease: Periungual desquamation in a 3-year-old on the 12th day of illness. (Reprinted with permission of the Council on Cardiovascular Disease in the Young, Committee on Rheumatic Fever, Endocarditis, and Kawasaki Disease, American Heart Association Diagnostic Guidelines for Kawasaki Disease. *Circulation.* 2001;103:335-336.)

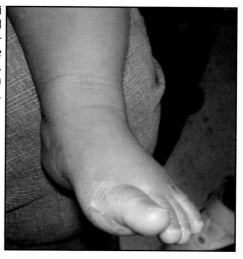

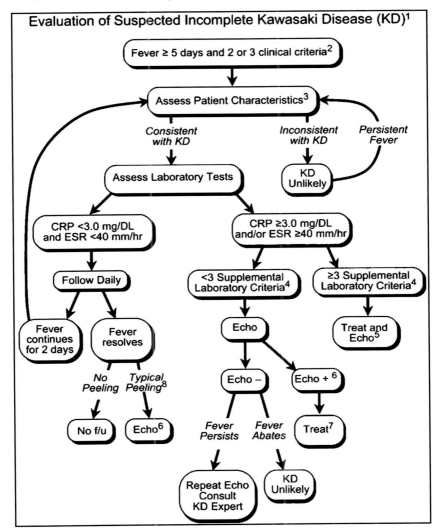

Figure 45-5. Algorithm for diagnosis of patients with incomplete Kawasaki disease (KD). Evaluation of suspected incomplete KD. (1) In the absence of a gold standard for diagnosis, this algorithm cannot be evidence-based but rather represents the informed opinion of the Expert Committee. Consultation with an expert should be sought anytime assistance is needed. (2) Infants 6 months old on day 7 of fever with no other explanation should undergo laboratory testing and, if evidence of systemic inflammation is found, echocardiography, even if the infants have no clinical criteria. (3) Characteristics suggesting disease other than KD include exudative conjunctivitis, exudative pharyngitis, discrete intraoral lesions, bullous or vesicular rash, or generalized adenopathy. Consider alternative diagnoses. (4) Supplemental laboratory criteria include albumin value of 3.0 g/dL (30.0 g/L), anemia for age, elevation of alanine aminotransferase, platelet count of more than $450.0 \times 10^3/\mu L$ ($450.0 \times 10^9/L$) after 7 days, white blood cell count $15.0 \times 10^3/\mu L$ ($15.0 \times 10^9/L$), and 10 white blood cells/high-power field in the urine. (5) Can treat before performing echocardiography (Echo). (6) Echocardiography is considered positive for purposes of this algorithm if any of 3 conditions are met: z score for left anterior descending or right coronary artery of 2.5; coronary arteries meet Japanese Ministry of Health criteria for aneurysms; or 3 other suggestive features exist, including perivascular brightness, lack of tapering, decreased left ventricular function, mitral regurgitation, pericardial effusion, or z scores in left anterior descending or right coronary artery of 2 to 2.5. (7) If echocardiography is positive, children should be treated within 10 days of fever onset and those beyond day 10 with clinical and laboratory signs (C-reactive protein, erythrocyte sedimentation rate) of ongoing inflammation. (8) Typical peeling begins under nail bed of fingers and then toes. (Reprinted with permission of Diagnosis, treatment, and long-term management of Kawasaki disease: a statement for health professionals from the Committee on Rheumatic Fever, Endocarditis, and Kawasaki Disease, Council on Cardiovascular Disease in the Young, American Heart Association. *Circulation.* 2004;110:1748.)

There are several other etiologies that may present with clinical signs and symptoms that are similar to KD, making this a more challenging scenario for diagnosis. Systemic juvenile idiopathic arthritis may be a consideration, particularly if the child has additional findings including involvement of 1 or more joints and systemic organ involvement. Drug hypersensitivity reactions may also manifest with many of these findings, but the rash may often consist of hives or erythema multiforme (discrete target lesions). In addition, Stevens-Johnson syndrome may be triggered by viral (herpes simplex virus) or bacterial (*Mycoplasma*) causes as well as medications (such as TMP-SMX and anticonvulsants). Often individuals present with fever, malaise, maculopapular rash (which may involve plaques) and mucosal involvement. Individuals tend to have a toxic or systemically ill appearance. Treatment is largely supportive, with topical agents to the skin and mucosa used to prevent secondary infection.

There are quite a few infectious diseases that may produce a clinical picture with some or all of the findings of KD and should be considered. Adenovirus may cause upper respiratory infection including pharyngitis, otitis media, tonsillitis, pharyngoconjunctival fever (most often with serotypes 3 and 7), and pneumonia. In older children, adenovirus is one of the most common causes of epidemic viral keratoconjunctivitis (usually due to serotypes 8, 19, and 37). Treatment and management is largely supportive, with strict hand hygiene to avoid transmission of the highly infectious conjunctivitis.

Measles (rubeola) is a febrile exanthem that may present with cough, coryza, conjunctivitis, Koplik spots (bluish spots with an erythematous base in the interior mucosa). The rash is a rather diffuse fulminant maculopapular exanthem. In the United States, due to routine vaccination, this diagnosis is less likely; however, it should be considered in individuals with recent travel to endemic areas, international adoptees, and/or children who are un- or under vaccinated. Treatment and management is largely supportive. Vitamin A is traditionally administered in developing countries or in vitamin A-deficient individuals, as it has been shown to reduce morbidity and mortality.

Epstein-Barr virus (EBV) is a common viral infection and often presents with fever, malaise, and an exudative pharyngitis. Individuals who have been administered antibiotics such as amoxicillin may experience a maculopapular rash. The viral illness may wax and wane, with nonspecific symptoms of fever, headache, and fatigue, sometimes for weeks to months. Treatment and management is largely supportive with the exception that individuals should be examined for splenomegaly, and if present, should be restricted from contact sports until resolution.

Group A beta hemolytic streptococcus infections due to more than 120 serotypes of *Streptococcus pyogenes* are common causes of febrile illness in school-aged children. Most characteristically, these infections cause an exudative pharyngitis, abdominal pain, and erythematous scarlatiniform ("sandpaper") rash, which may present an overall toxic appearance. The rash tends to begin in the neck area and later be detected on the anterior and posterior trunk. Treatment with oral penicillin is the drug of choice to prevent rheumatic heart disease but does not decrease the possibility of poststreptococcal glomerulonephritis.

Rocky Mountain spotted fever should be a consideration, particularly in children with a history of a potential tick bite, but may present with the classic triad of fever, headache, and rash. The rash tends to be petechial and initially is often detected at the hands and feet and later occurs at other body locations. Other features include nausea, vomiting, anorexia, myalgias, and abdominal pain. Diagnostics may reveal hyponatremia and

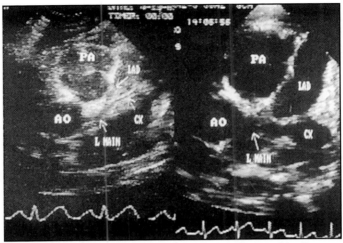

Figure 45-6. Clinical manifestations of Kawasaki disease: Two-dimensional echocardiogram. AO = indicates aorta; CX = circumflex coronary; LAD = left anterior descending coronary; L Main = left main coronary; and PA = pulmonary artery. (Reprinted with permission of the Council on Cardiovascular Disease in the Young, Committee on Rheumatic Fever, Endocarditis, and Kawasaki Disease, American Heart Association Diagnostic Guidelines for Kawasaki Disease. *Circulation*. 2001;103;335-336.)

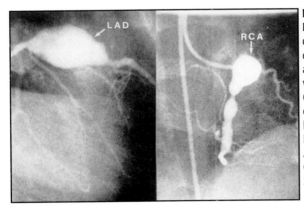

Figure 45-7. Clinical manifestations of Kawasaki disease: Coronary angiogram demonstrating hugely dilated left anterior descending (LAD) artery with obstruction and very dilated right coronary artery (RCA) with an area of severe narrowing in a 6-year-old boy. (Reprinted with permission of the Council on Cardiovascular Disease in the Young, Committee on Rheumatic Fever, Endocarditis, and Kawasaki Disease, American Heart Association Diagnostic Guidelines for Kawasaki Disease. *Circulation*. 2001;103;335-336.)

thrombocytopenia. Symptoms may last several weeks and may have severe end-organ disease, disseminated intravascular coagulation (DIC), and death. Treatment is generally empiric doxycycline (regardless of age).

It is prudent to investigate the possibility of the above-mentioned causes for this clinical scenario, as elimination of these possibilities allows for a more prompt diagnosis of KD and thus prompt definitive treatment. IVIG should be administered within the first 10 days of fever, along with high-dose aspirin in order to decrease the known sequelae of aneurysms, myocardial infarction, and sudden death (Figures 45-6 and 45-7). If there is suspicion of KD given clinical examination findings, consultation with a specialist in pediatric infectious diseases and/or pediatric cardiologist is advised, as children with a diagnosis of KD are followed after their initial treatment course to monitor for later development of coronary artery abnormalities.

Suggested Readings

American Academy of Pediatrics. Pickering LK, Baker CJ, Kimberlin DW, Long SS, eds. *Red Book: 2009 Report of the Committee on Infectious Diseases.* 28th ed. Elk Gove Village, IL: American Academy of Pediatrics; 2009.

Newburger JW, Takahashi M, Gerber MA, et al. Diagnosis, treatment, and long-term management of Kawasaki disease: a statement for health professionals from the Committee on Rheumatic Fever, Endocarditis, and Kawasaki Disease, Council on Cardiovascular Disease in the Young, American Heart Association. *Pediatrics.* 2004;114(6):1708-1733.

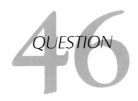

WHAT IMAGING EVALUATION SHOULD I CONSIDER IN AN 11-YEAR-OLD MALE WITH A 2-WEEK HISTORY OF FEVER AND COMPLAINTS OF LOW BACK PAIN AND A PROGRESSIVE LIMP?

Laura Patricia Stadler, MEd, MD, MS

This clinical scenario is concerning for an infectious process involving the vertebral bodies (osteomyelitis) and/or intervertebral disk spaces (discitis). In addition, a malignant process should be ruled out of the differential diagnosis. These clinical entities are uncommon in children but can be significant illnesses with substantial morbidity and mortality. It is thought that a preceding infection (whether bacteremia from organisms such as *Staphylococcus aureus*, *Streptococcus pyogenes*, *Streptococcus pneumoniae* or GI/GU pathogens such as *Escherichia coli*) may hematogenously spread to the vertebral bodies and/or disk spaces.

Although both entities may present with these clinical signs and symptoms, an 18-year review of discitis and vertebral osteomyelitis in children indicated that children with discitis were usually younger than 5 years with no or low-grade fever. Refusal to walk occurred secondary to a lesion usually in the lumbar area. However, children with osteomyelitis tended to be older and have fever and pain in cervical, thoracic, or lumbar regions. When suspicious of either of these infectious processes, it is important to define the anatomy and extent of disease for prognosis, appropriate intervention, determination of the microbiology, treatment, and management.

The initial studies one may order consist of plain x-rays of the spine. Most authorities believe changes consistent with a diagnosis of osteomyelitis (such as periosteal elevation and bony destruction) will not be present for 7 to 10 days and discitis approximately 2 to 3 weeks. Figure 46-1A and B shows bony destruction of the L4-L5 vertebral bodies of a 9-month-old child with a history of refusal to sit up and bear weight coupled with fever for 2 weeks. In the pediatric population, Fernandez et al indicate that roughly three-fourths of patients with discitis had abnormalities detected via plain films.

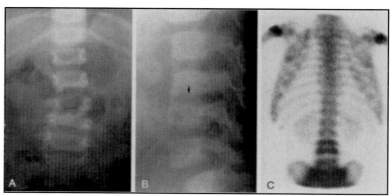

Figure 46-1. (A) Frontal and (B) lateral radiographs of lumbar spine show narrowing of L3-L4 intervertebral disk space with irregularity of the adjacent vertebral end plate (arrow). (C) Radioisotope bone scan shows increased activity at L3 and L4 levels.

Other imaging modalities such as nuclear bone scan and computed tomography (CT) scan are relatively nonspecific. Figure 46-1C shows the aforementioned 9-month-old with enhancement in the lower lumbar vertebral bodies, but it is difficult to determine the extent of disease, the consistency of the abnormality present, and the anatomic landmarks. Although one of these diagnostic modalities may be abnormal, it may require that an additional study be performed to better delineate the clinical scenario.

Magnetic resonance imaging (MRI) with contrast has become the imaging diagnostic of choice in order to define the anatomy and pathology of the central nervous system, vertebral bodies, and intervertebral spaces, as well as the musculoskeletal areas in which there may be local extension of disease. MRI is widely available, and an additional advantage to this procedure is the potential ability to perform image-guided sampling (needle biopsy) for both diagnostic and therapeutic purposes. Some considerations prior to MRI include sedation of young infants and/or children and whether a contraindication to the contrast exists.

Figure 46-2 shows a T2-weighted image of a child's upper thoracic spine demonstration of osteomyelitis with destruction of a vertebral body, and discitis. In addition, arrows indicate a paraspinous phlegmon and/or hemorrhage.

Although plain films may initially be performed to evaluate for the presence of trauma or lytic lesions, MRI is often utilized for definitive diagnosis. In the pediatric review, of 13 patients with vertebral osteomyelitis, only 46% of plain films were abnormal, indicating that MRI may be necessary for detection such that treatment and management may be given. In general, MRI was the recommended imaging modality of choice for pediatric infections of the spine, as 9 of 10 patients with discitis and 11 of 11 children with vertebral osteomyelitis were detected by MRI.

The most common organism detected by biopsy is *S aureus*, with methicillin-resistant *S aureus* (MRSA) comprising a significant portion of isolates. Other organisms include *S pyogenes*, *S pneumoniae*, and gram-negative organisms (*E coli*) associated with a prior history of urinary tract infections. *Bartonella henselae* is an uncommon cause of vertebral osteomyelitis, but should be considered in individuals with cat exposure. Lastly, *Mycobacterium*

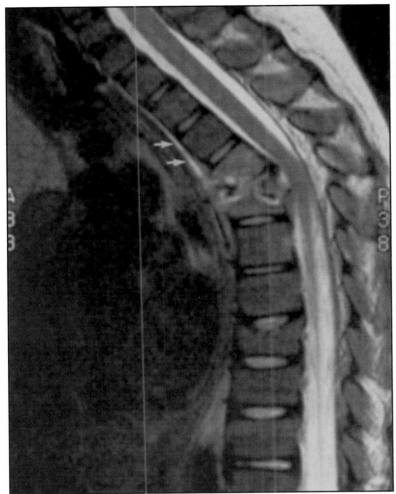

Figure 46-2. T2-weighted image of the upper thoracic spine demonstrating osteomyelitis, with destruction of the vertebral body, and discitis. The white arrows define a thin band of high signal intensity in the anterior spinal tissues, representing a paraspinous phlegmon and/or a small collection of hemorrhage. Despite this degree of apparent destruction and spinal cord edema, no neurologic symptoms or signs were noted. (Reproduced with permission of *Pediatrics*, Vol. 105, Pages 1299-1304, Copyright © 2006 by the AAP.)

tuberculosis, or "Pott disease" (spondylitis more commonly affecting the cervical and thoracic vertebrae), may be suspected in patients with a positive TB skin test (TST), interferon gamma release assay (IGRA), and/or associated tuberculosis (TB) risk factors.

Given the broad differential, it is crucial to obtain microbiologic identification and susceptibilities to guide antimicrobial therapy. If cultures remain negative, options for management include a repeat biopsy or empiric anti-staphylococcal therapy. If the local epidemiology suggests the percentage of MRSA is significant, consideration of vancomycin or clindamycin is reasonable. Other anti-staphylococcal drugs targeting methicillin-susceptible *S aureus* include nafcillin, oxacillin, or cefazolin. Clindamycin may be a prudent choice as it provides empiric coverage of both staphylococci and streptococci, with the added benefit of bone penetration.

The proposed length of therapy is unknown, but generally a minimum of 4 to 6 weeks with clinical improvement, normalization of inflammatory markers (such as erythrocyte sedimentation rate [ESR], C reactive protein [CRP]), +/– repeat imaging used for determining duration of antibiotics.

Suggested Readings

Fernandez M, Carrol C, Baker CJ. Discitis and vertebral osteomyelitis in children: an 18 year review. *Pediatrics.* 2000; 105(6):1299-1304.

Mahboubi S, Morris MC. Imaging of spinal infections in children. *Radiol Clin North Am.* 2001;39(2):215-222.

SECTION XV

CANDIDIASIS

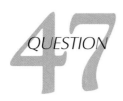

A 5-WEEK-OLD INFANT WAS RECENTLY DIAGNOSED WITH THRUSH AND TREATED WITH NYSTATIN FOR 10 DAYS WITHOUT IMPROVEMENT. SHOULD I OBTAIN A CULTURE OF THE INFANT'S MUCOSA AND CHANGE HIS THERAPY? WHAT OTHER PROBLEMS SHOULD I BE THINKING ABOUT IN THIS SETTING?

Amber Hoffman, MD

Candida species are the most common cause of oropharyngeal fungal infections, or thrush, in infants. *Candida albicans* accounts for the vast majority of thrush. The skin, gastrointestinal tract, and respiratory tract of neonates become colonized with microbial flora within the first months of life. Vaginal deliveries are thought to introduce infant colonization of the rectum and skin with *Candida sp.* Between 25% and 33% of pregnant women have *C albicans* in their vaginal flora, and close to a third of these women are asymptomatic. Introduction of bacterial and fungal colonization can also occur from breast-feeding, bottle nipples, or pacifiers that have been improperly cleaned or have been in another person's mouth. Hand contact, or even kissing, can also transmit *C albicans* from mothers to infants. Low birth weight infants are at a higher risk for fungal colonization as well. Beyond the neonatal period, *C albicans* is considered to be part of a normal oral and intestinal flora, which is typically kept in balance by other microbes.[1]

Oral candidiasis peaks in the fourth week of life with a prevalence of around 14%. Once appearing in the mouth, *Candida* organisms appear in the feces approximately 2 to 3 days later, where they can also cause diaper dermatitis. Thrush occurs in 1% to 37% of healthy infants, and if left untreated, it will generally resolve in 3 to 8 weeks. When thrush causes poor feeding or discomfort due to mucositis or esophagitis, treatment with medication can hasten the resolution of the infection and improve the infant's symptoms.[1]

The first step in evaluating a "treatment failure" is to repeat a history and a physical examination. Once focused on the diagnosis of thrush, caregivers, parents, and childcare providers may think that the appearance of formula, or breast milk, on the tongue represents thrush. If it can be easily wiped away without revealing an erythematous, or erosive mucosa, then the child does not likely have clinical thrush. The "treatment failure" may be a nonrecognition that the illness has resolved and a misidentification of breast milk or formula on the tongue.

The physical examination and history should also extend beyond the infant's symptomatology to address proper cleansing of bottle nipples and pacifiers as well as breastfeeding practices, as both may lead to reinnoculation and subsequent reinfection. Mothers who have yeast around their nipples may reinnoculate the infant during breast-feeding unless the mother is treated as well.[2] Signs and symptoms of a candidal infection in a breast-feeding mother can be variable, which can make the diagnosis challenging. The nipple and areola may be more pink, red, or purple than usual. There may be flaking of the skin on the nipple or areola or satellite lesions. The mother may have no rash but have nipple pain, itching, or a deep, dagger-like pain in the breast. This pain may be worse with, or immediately after, breast-feeding. If the mother appears to have only superficial skin findings, then a topical antifungal cream may be effective. Deeper breast pain is an indication for systemic therapy such as oral fluconazole. If using the mother's breast symptoms as the primary reason for treating the infant, one must consider nonfungal breast pathology such as eczema, mastitis, impetigo, psoriasis, nipple trauma from inappropriate latching, or other chronic forms of dermatitis.[2]

Physicians who have been polled regarding their practice patterns for initial treatment of thrush in the breast-feeding dyad reported starting with topical nystatin cream for the mother and nystatin solution for the infant, followed by oral fluconazole for the mother and nystatin solution for the infant, followed by oral fluconazole for both. For thrush recurrence, the most common regimens were oral nystatin for the infant and nystatin cream for the mother followed by oral fluconazole for both the mother and infant.[2]

Early studies suggested that nystatin had between an 80% and 90% treatment success, which made it a mainstay of therapy for decades. Nystatin is also relatively inexpensive with a low adverse effect profile, making it a desirable first-line agent. A more recent study indicates that the clinical cure rate is closer to 54% in healthy infants. Some of this may be due to poor adherence of the solution to the oral mucosa, which is why gels have been tried. Newer antifungal medications have emerged on the market that have been studied in both immunocompetent and immunocompromised patients who appear to have higher clinical cure rates but also come with higher monetary costs and different side effect profiles.[3]

In the 1950s and 1960s, gentian violet and amphotericin B were compared with nystatin. Cure rates at that time were reported to be around 75% for gentian violet and 80% for amphotericin B. Gentian violet stains mucous membranes and skin temporarily. It can also stain clothing. More important than staining though is that it can cause irritation, vesicles, and ulcerations. When used in the mouth, it can lead to esophagitis, laryngitis, tracheitis, or a severe mucositis, which are undesirable adverse events that may be worse than the thrush symptoms. Amphotericin B is more commonly used in its IV form to treat severe systemic fungal infections rather than for oral thrush in healthy infants.[3]

Other antifungal medications that have been evaluated include clotrimazole, in the form of a cream as well as an oral troche, and miconazole gel. Miconazole has been compared with nystatin suspension and nystatin gel. The clinical cure rate for miconazole gel compared to nystatin gel on day 8 was 96.9% versus 37.6% and by day 12 was 99% versus 54.1%. However, neither of these medication formulations is readily available in the United States.[4]

Fluconazole is readily available in the United States and can easily be given orally. The clinical cure rate with fluconazole has been found to be as high as 100% with 7 days of therapy compared to 28.6% with 10 days of nystatin therapy. Microbiologic cure was reported as 73.3% and 5.6%, respectively. Recurrence of clinical disease was evaluated in the fluconazole-treated group only. Clinical relapse was 23% by day 28 after therapy was initiated and 56% had microbiologic recurrence.[4]

In the studies that include microbiologic cultures to evaluate for fungal eradication and recurrence in immunocompetent hosts, the vast majority of yeast continues to be *C albicans*. Non-albicans yeasts included *Candida parapsilosis*, *Candida lusitaniae*, *Candida famata*, and *Candida pulcherrima*. Given the low rate of resistance, even in immunocompromised hosts when it comes to oral candidiasis,[5] there is not a significant role for culture in an immunocompetent host. Clinical cures are higher than microbial cures in multiple studies, and the presence of the yeast does not indicate that there will be a clinical relapse. Keep in mind that *C albicans* is considered part of the normal flora and its presence in the absence of clinical disease is to be expected.[4]

In the case of refractory or recurrent thrush, or thrush that appears in the first week of life, the history and physical examination must concentrate on looking for an underlying reason such as an immunodeficiency rather than turning to cultures. Fungal infection can be the presenting sign in a child with a T-cell–mediated immunodeficiency, such as human immunodeficiency virus (HIV), severe combined immunodeficiency, and hyper-IgM syndrome. Other signs and symptoms for T-cell–mediated primary immunodeficiency are recurrent diarrheal illnesses, failure to thrive, malabsorption, and chronic respiratory symptoms.[6]

Infants who are receiving antibiotics or corticosteroids may be predisposed to developing thrush. It can be more difficult to eradicate oral candidiasis in these patients until those medications are stopped. The mother may also be predisposed to developing cutaneous candidiasis of her breasts if she is taking one of these medications or if she has a medical condition such as diabetes that predisposes her to fungal illness. If on examination the child indeed has white plaques on the buccal, gingival, or lingual mucosa, and the caregivers have appropriately implemented external control measures, such as bottle/pacifier cleansing/replacement and/or treatment for the breast-feeding mother, then consideration should be given to changing therapy rather than repeating the course with additional education.

Overall, the take home message is that thrush is very common, especially in a 5-week-old infant. There appears to be a high failure rate with nystatin, but given its low cost and low adverse drug event profile, it remains a desirable first-line option. Assessment of environmental factors should be considered part of the therapy (ie, addressing maternal infection, bottle and pacifier cleaning, and hand hygiene). If these additional areas were not addressed in the first treatment regimen, then one could consider implementing them and repeating the course. Given the high failure rate of nystatin, one could also try a course of fluconazole. There is not a significant role for culture, except in the known immunodeficient host with prolonged, recurrent courses of antifungal medications.

Also, an immunodeficiency evaluation should not be considered in a child who has failed one course of nystatin unless there is a significant history of immune-deficiency in the family, HIV risk factors, or the child has other signs and symptoms of immune deficiency such as failure to thrive, diarrhea, malabsorption, or recurrent infections.

References

1. Hoppe, JE. Treatment of oropharyngeal candidiasis and candidal diaper dermatitis in neonates and infants: review and reappraisal. *The Pediatric Infectious Disease Journal.* 1997;19(9):885-894.
2. Hoppe, JE. Treatment of Oropharyngeal Candidiasis in Immunocompetent Infants: a Randomized Multicenter Study of Miconazole Gel vs. Nystatin Suspension. *The Pediatric Infectious Disease Journal.* 1997;16(3):288-293.
3. Brent NB. Thrush in the breastfeeding dyad: results of a survey on diagnosis and treatment. *Clin Pediatr.* 2001;40(9):503-506.
4. Goins RA. Comparison of fluconazole and nystatin oral suspensions for treatment of oral candidiasis in infants. *The Pediatric Infectious Disease J.* 2002;21(12):1165-1167.
5. Darouiche RO. Oropharyngeal and esophageal candidiasis in immunocompromised patients: treatment issues. *Clin Infect Dis* 1998;26(2):259-274.
6. Fuleihan R. Immunology. In: *Nelson Essentials of Pediatrics.* 5th ed. 2006;72:363-369.

SECTION XVI

RECURRENT FEVER

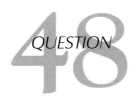

WHAT DIAGNOSTIC TESTING, IF ANY, SHOULD BE PERFORMED FOR A NORMALLY DEVELOPING TODDLER WHO ATTENDS A DAY CARE CENTER, DEVELOPS FREQUENT FEVERS, AND COMMONLY HAS RESPIRATORY TRACT SYMPTOMS? WHAT IS THE MOST COMMON REASON FOR THIS PRESENTATION?

Aimee Hersh, MD and Erica F. Lawson, MD

The most common cause of recurrent fevers and respiratory tract symptoms in children who attend day care centers is recurrent infections. Modes of transmission of infection in day care centers include respiratory, fecal-oral, as well as direct and indirect (fomite) contact with bodily fluids. The ages and health status of children and caregivers, hygiene practices, and the condition of the facility all influence exposure to pathogens. Common respiratory viruses found in childcare centers include respiratory syncytial virus, para-influenza, rhinoviruses, human metapneumoviruses, coronaviruses, and influenza. *Bordetella pertussis*, *Streptococcus pneumoniae*, *Haemophilus influenzae*, and varicella zoster virus are other common respiratory pathogens.[1]

Most children with recurrent infections will not have any underlying abnormality, and do not require additional diagnostic testing. Children have a median of 5 colds per year, but more than 10% of children will have 10 or more colds per year. A healthy child should clear infections completely. The mean duration of viral cold symptoms is 8 days but may be longer than 2 weeks. Asymptomatic periods between infections are expected. Growth and development should remain normal.[2]

When should you worry that a patient with frequent respiratory infections could have an underlying chronic condition? The acronym "SPUR" is a useful mnemonic.

- Severe infection
- Persistent infection
- Unusual organisms or complications
- Recurrent infection

Acute and chronic otitis media are among the most common recurrent infections of childhood and may become problematic even in otherwise healthy children. The average child will have 1 to 2 episodes of otitis media per year. Repeated courses of antibiotics can breed resistant organisms, making otitis increasingly difficult to treat. Tympanostomy tube placement should be considered for children who develop 5 or more infections per year, infections resistant to antibiotics, or hearing loss. Immunodeficiency should be considered if the child has more than 8 episodes of otitis media per year, especially in the presence of other recurrent infections.

About 30% of children with recurrent infections will have atopic disease. A child with allergic rhinitis and asthma may have chronic respiratory symptoms misdiagnosed as recurrent infections and may also be at increased risk for secondary infections such as otitis media, acute or chronic sinusitis, and bacterial pneumonia. Patients with persistent symptoms may benefit from referral to an allergist.

Chronic diseases such as cystic fibrosis, congenital heart disease, or chronic aspiration are identified in 10% of children with recurrent infections. These patients often present with failure to thrive, chronic respiratory symptoms, and physical examination findings such as clubbing or barrel chest. Referral to a pulmonologist is appropriate for a child with chronic pulmonary symptoms that do not resolve between infections.

Finally, 10% of children with recurrent infections will have an immunodeficiency. Immunodeficiency may be primary (congenital) or secondary (acquired). Secondary immunodeficiencies may be due to HIV, underlying malignancy, immunosuppressant medications, diabetes mellitus, and many other conditions. Careful history and physical examination will often reveal clues to the presence of an underlying condition, which predisposed the patient to recurrent infections.

Red flags for a primary immunodeficiency include the following[3]:

- More than 10 new infections within 12 months
- Two or more episodes of severe sinusitis or bacterial pneumonia in 1 year
- Two or more months on antibiotics without improvement in symptoms
- Failure to thrive
- Recurrent abscesses of the skin or organs
- Thrush after the age of 1 year
- Complications after live vaccinations
- Need for IV antibiotics to clear infections
- Opportunistic or invasive infections
- Family history of primary immunodeficiency

Table 48-1
Initial Evaluation of the Immune System

	Humoral Immunity	*Cell-mediated Immunity*
Quantitative measurements	IgA, IgM, IgE, IgG IgG$_1$, IgG$_2$, IgG$_3$, IgG$_4$	T cells (CD3+, CD4+, CD8+) B cells (CD19+) NK cells (CD16+, CD56+)
Functional measurements	Pneumococcal antibodies Tetanus antibodies	Mitogen stimulation testing* Antigen stimulation testing*

*These tests are not typically performed as a part of the initial primary immunodeficiency evaluation.

Which primary immunodeficiency to suspect depends on several factors, including the age and gender of the patient and the types of infections seen.[4] Infants less than 6 months who present with recurrent fevers and severe respiratory infections are more likely to have a T-cell immunodeficiency, such as severe combined immunodeficiency (SCID) or CD40 ligand deficiency. In older infants and toddlers, recurrent sinobacterial infection is suggestive of a humoral immunodeficiency, such as common variable immunodeficiency or x-linked agammaglobulinemia.

The initial evaluation of the immune system can be divided into defects in humoral or cell-mediated immunity, as well as quantitative or functional defects (Table 48-1).

When primary immunodeficiency is suspected, investigation should begin with a complete blood count with differential. Cell counts should be evaluated, with attention to absolute numbers of lymphocytes and neutrophils. Lymphocyte subset analysis should also be obtained, looking at absolute numbers of CD3+, CD4+, CD8+, B lymphocytes (CD19+, CD20+), and natural killer (NK) cells (CD16+, CD56+). Serum immunoglobulins should be measured, including IgA, IgM, IgE, IgG, and IgG subclasses. Specific antibody responses to tetanus and pneumococcal vaccines should be measured. Immune response is expected within 4 weeks of first exposure to vaccine, although pneumococcal serologies must be matched to those present in either the pneumococcal 13-valent vaccine (1, 3, 4, 5, 6A, 6B, 7F, 9V, 14, 18C, 19A, 19F, and 23F) or the 23-valent vaccine (1, 2, 3, 4, 5, 6B, 7F, 8, 9N, 9V, 10A, 11A, 12F, 14, 15B, 17F, 18C, 19F, 19A, 20, 22F, 23F, 33F). Presence of tetanus antibodies signifies the capability to respond to antigens with a T-cell–dependent antibody response. Presence of pneumococcal antibodies after vaccination with the 13-valent vaccine signifies the ability to respond to protein conjugated polysaccharides with a T-cell–associated B-cell response. In order to define a pure B-cell response, some experts recommend obtaining serology before and after 23-valent unconjugated polysaccharide pneumococcal vaccine, which measures the ability to respond to polysaccharide antigens independent of T cells. Referral to an immunologist is appropriate for any patient with a suspected primary immunodeficiency.

References

1. Mink CM, Yeh S. Infections in child-care facilities and schools. *Pediatr Rev.* 2009;30(7):259-269.
2. Bush A. Recurrent respiratory infections. *Pediatr Clin North Am.* 2009;56(1):67-100.
3. Jeffrey Moddell foundation web site accessed on: September 10, 2011.
   http://www.info4pi.org/aboutPI/index.cfm?section=aboutPI&content=warningsigns&CFID=72617&CFTOKEN=48700864
4. Slatter MA, Gennery AR. Clinical immunology review series: an approach to the patient with recurrent infections in childhood. *Clin Exp Immunol.* 2008;152(3):389-396.
5. Balmer P, Cant AJ, Borrow R. Anti-pneumococcal antibody titre measurement: what useful information does it yield? *J Clin Pathol.* 2007;60(4):345-350.

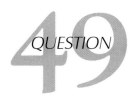

A 2-Year-Old Patient Has Had Recurrent Fevers for the Last Year. He Often Has a Red Throat, Adenopathy, and Stomatitis With His Fevers. I Am Concerned About Periodic Fever, Aphthous Stomatitis, Pharyngitis, and Cervical Adenitis Syndrome. What Are the Treatment Options for This Diagnosis?

Aimee Hersh, MD and Erica F. Lawson, MD

Periodic fever, aphthous stomatitis, pharyngitis, and cervical adenitis (PFAPA) syndrome, is the most common periodic fever syndrome of childhood. The diagnosis of a periodic fever syndrome should be considered in a child who has a history of recurrent episodes of fever, occurring at predictable (periodic) time intervals, and when more common causes of fever, such as recurrent or chronic infection, have been excluded.

There are several clues in the history that can help distinguish a periodic fever syndrome from recurrent or chronic infection. First, the febrile episodes of periodic fever syndromes tend to be predictable, occurring at regular intervals. Symptoms that accompany the fevers are generally the same from episode to episode. In the case of PFAPA, the most common symptoms are aphthous stomatitis (painful oral ulcers), pharyngitis (red and painful posterior oropharynx with tonsillar enlargement), and cervical adenitis (tender anterior cervical lymphadenopathy). Secondly, one of the hallmarks of a periodic fever syndrome is a complete lack of symptoms and a normal physical examination between episodes of fever, which is generally not true in the case of an underlying chronic infectious or inflammatory process. Similarly, inflammatory markers erythrocyte sedimentation rate (ESR), C-reactive protein (CRP) tend to rise during the fever episodes and

Table 49-1

Characteristics of the Genetic Periodic Fever Syndromes

	Gene	*Clinical Characteristics*	*Fever Interval*	*Duration of Fever Episode*
Familial Mediterranean fever (FMF)	MEFV	Fever with serositis, arthritis, erysipelas-like rash	Weeks to months	12 to 72 hours
Tumor necrosis factor receptor-associated periodic syndrome (TRAPS)	TNFRSF 1A	Fever with localized muscle pain, conjunctivitis, periorbital edema, and rash	Weeks to months	1 to 2 weeks
Hyperimm-unoglobulin D syndrome (HIDS)	MVK	Fever with cervical adenitis, abdominal pain, vomiting and diarrhea; symptoms can be provoked with trauma	4 to 6 weeks	4 to 6 days
Cyclic neutropenia	ELA2	Fevers with recurrent bacterial infections	18 to 24 days	3 days
Familial Cold Autoinflammatory syndrome (FCAS)	NOD2/CARD 15	Urticaria, arthralgias, and conjunctivitis after cold exposure	Intermittent	Days
Muckle-Wells syndrome	NOD2/CARD 15	Urticaria, arthralgias, and conjunctivitis not associated with cold. Can cause deafness	Intermittent	Days
Neonatal-onset multisystem inflammatory disorder (NOMID)	NOD2/CARD 15	Rash, arthropathy with growth impairment, aseptic meningitis with progressive CNS impairment	Intermittent	Days

then normalize once the fever resolves. If the inflammatory markers remain elevated between fever episodes, then a diagnosis other than a periodic fever syndrome should be considered.

Once the fever pattern is felt to be consistent with a periodic fever syndrome, other elements of the history and physical examination may help pinpoint a specific syndrome. The interval between fevers, duration of the fever episodes, typical symptoms (eg, mouth sores, rash, arthritis) family history and ethnicity are all potentially important clues to identifying the specific periodic fever syndrome (Table 49-1).[1]

The various periodic fever syndromes have overlapping symptoms; therefore, a definitive diagnosis of PFAPA cannot be made until other periodic fever syndromes have been excluded via genetic testing, which can be done via GeneDx (www.genedx.com).

PFAPA typically presents in children younger than 5 years. The typical patient has 3 to 6 days of high fevers (38.9°C to 41.1°C), which on average occurs every 30 days. Criteria for diagnosis include the presence of recurrent, predictable episodes of high fever accompanied by at least 1 of the 3 major clinical findings associated with PFAPA (aphthous stomatitis, pharyngitis, or lymphadenitis), a well interval between episodes, and the exclusion of another cause of recurrent fever.[2]

In general, PFAPA is felt to be a benign and self-limited disease. Patients with PFAPA have normal growth and development, and there does not appear to be any residual sequelae from PFAPA after symptoms resolve. Most patients with PFAPA will outgrow the condition by 10 years of age; however, the mean duration of symptoms is approximately 4.5 years. The frequency and severity of the fever episodes vary from patient to patient, but for many the episodes can be disruptive and impair their ability to participate in regular activities, including school. For this reason, many families chose to pursue treatment for PFAPA.

There are several treatment options for PFAPA. For symptomatic management, regular dosing of ibuprofen and acetaminophen during fever episodes can reduce the height of the fever and also lessen the pain associated with aphthous stomatitis and pharyngitis.

Another treatment option is corticosteroids. The majority of patients will experience a dramatic resolution of fever within 2 to 24 hours with a single dose of prednisone or prednisolone (1 to 2 mg/kg, maximum dose of 60 mg) at the start of a fever episode. This dose can be repeated every 12 hours for up to 3 total doses if the fever persists. Families should be aware that approximately 25% to 50% of patients will experience a shortening by 1 to 2 weeks of the interval between fever episodes when prednisone is used.

Cimetidine is used as a prophylactic medication to prevent fever episodes. The typical dose is 20 to 40 mg/kg/d, with a maximum dose of 150 mg twice daily. Approximately 25% of patients will experience a remission of PFAPA symptoms with cimetidine; some patients who respond to cimetidine will experience a recurrence of symptoms once the cimetidine is discontinued.

Tonsillectomy has emerged as a potentially curative treatment for PFAPA. Although the cause of PFAPA is unknown, the high rate of pharyngitis suggests that chronically inflamed lymphoid tissue may be the stimulus for recurrent inflammatory episodes. The theory is that surgical removal of this tissue eliminates the inflammatory stimulus and prevents further fever episodes. There have been 2 recent randomized control trials and several observational studies that support the use of tonsillectomy for treatment of PFAPA. If a patient is considering tonsillectomy, the risks and benefits of surgery, balanced with the natural history of PFAPA and the medical options for treatment, need to be considered carefully.[3]

References

1. Feder HM, Salazar JC. A clinical review of 105 patients with PFAPA (a periodic fever syndrome). *Acta Paediatr.* 2010;99(2):178-184.
2. Caorsi R, Pelagatti MA, Federici S, Finetti M, Martini A, Gattorno M. Periodic fever, apthous stomatitis, pharyngitis and adenitis syndrome. *Curr Opin Rheumatol.* 2010;22(5):579-584.
3. Burton MJ, Pollard AJ, Ramsden JD. Tonsillectomy for periodic fever, aphthous stomatitis, pharyngitis and cervical adenitis syndrome (PFAPA). The Cochrane Collaboration. *Cochrane Database Syst Rev.* 2010;(9):CD008669.

FINANCIAL DISCLOSURES

Dr. Susan Abdel-Rahman has no financial or proprietary interest in the materials presented herein.

Dr. Rebecca C. Brady has no financial or proprietary interest in the materials presented herein.

Dr. Christopher R. Cannavino has no financial or proprietary interest in the materials presented herein.

Dr. Archana Chatterjee receives a grant/research for GSK, MedImmune, Merck, Novartis, Pfizer, and Sanofi-Pasteur and is on the speaker's bureau/advisory board for GSK, MedImmune, Merck, Novartis, and Sanofi-Pasteur.

Dr. Ankhi Dutta has no financial or proprietary interest in the materials presented herein.

Dr. Jennifer Goldman has no financial or proprietary interest in the materials presented herein.

Dr. Christopher J. Harrison is a principal investigator for a MMR vaccine study.

Dr. Adam L. Hersh has no financial or proprietary interest in the materials presented herein.

Dr. Aimee Hersh has no financial or proprietary interest in the materials presented herein.

Dr. Amber Hoffman has no financial or proprietary interest in the materials presented herein.

Dr. Preeti Jaggi has no financial or proprietary interest in the materials presented herein.

Dr. Erica F. Lawson has no financial or proprietary interest in the materials presented herein.

Dr. Kimberly C. Martin has no financial or proprietary interest in the materials presented herein.

Dr. Angela L. Myers has no financial or proprietary interest in the materials presented herein.

Dr. Debra L. Palazzi has no financial or proprietary interest in the materials presented herein.

Dr. José R. Romero has no financial or proprietary interest in the materials presented herein.

Dr. Masako Shimamura has no financial or proprietary interest in the materials presented herein.

Dr. Kevin B. Spicer has no financial or proprietary interest in the materials presented herein.

Dr. Laura Patricia Stadler has no financial or proprietary interest in the materials presented herein.

Dr. Emily A. Thorell has no financial or proprietary interest in the materials presented herein.

Dr. Rene VanDeVoorde has no financial or proprietary interest in the materials presented herein.

Dr. Rebecca W. Widener has no financial or proprietary interest in the materials presented herein.

INDEX

acute gastroenteritis (AGE), 153
acute otitis media (AOM), 87, 101–105
  amoxicillin, 169
    works for, 102–103
  clindamycin, 89, 104
  drugs of choice for, 90
  MDR pneumococcus
    treatment of, 102–104
  oral cephalosporins, 103, 104
  parenteral ceftriaxone, 103–104
  pathogen among, 87
  serotype 19A, 104
acute respiratory distress syndrome, 65
adenopathy, 205
adenovirus, 153, 154, 162, 218
afebrile pneumonia syndrome of infancy, 81
  classic symptoms, 81
  nasopharyngeal specimen for culture, 82
  radiographic findings, 82
AGE. See gastroenteritis, acute
airway obstruction, 186
Alice-in-Wonderland syndrome, 186
alopecia areata, 47
Amblyomma americanum, 61
American Academy of Pediatrics (AAP)
  guidelines, 169
American dog ticks. See Dermacentor variabilis
amoxicillin, 18, 24, 71, 87–90, 93
  for acute bacterial adenitis, 211
  allergy, 88
  for AOM, 88–90
  with clavulanate, 24, 170, 177
  for early disseminated and late lyme
    disease, 73
  high-dose, 176
  resistance in nasopharyngeal flora, 170

  susceptibility of S pneumoniae to, 103
  for suspected bacterial CAP, 176
  for urinary tract infection prophylaxis, 18
amoxicillin-clavulanate, formulations of, 166
amphotericin B, 228
anaerobic bacteria, causing lymphadenitis,
  210, 212
anaplasmosis, 59, 61, 66
antibiotics
  for CA-MRSA abscesses, 24
  management of abscesses in children, 23
  recommended dosing for UTI, 18
  resistance, 176
    additional therapies, child with diarrhea, 151
  Salmonella typhi, treatments, 148
antimicrobial therapy, 205
  "aural toilet" to, 98
  microbiologic identification, and susceptibilities
    to guide, 223
  principles, 123
AOM. See acute otitis media (AOM)
Aspergillus species, 98
atopic dermatitis, 27, 28, 47
atypical pneumonia, 77
  causes of, 78
  clinical signs, 78
  diagnosis, 78
  pathogens associated with, 78
  symptoms, 77, 78
azithromycin, 205
  in AOM episode, 88
  in Babesiosis, 68
  in cat scratch disease, 205–207
  with erythromycin, 114, 148
  in pediatric patients with diarrhea, 148
  for penicillin-allergic patient, 114

resistance, 148
  for traveler's diarrhea, 151
  treating MDR 19A *S pneumoniae* with, 93

Babesia microti, 62, 68
babesiosis, 59
  antimicrobials for, 68
    dosages, 68
  causative agents, 62
  characteristics of, 62
  diagnosis, 62
  period of illness, 62
bacterial gastroenteritis, 149, 150. *See also* diarrhea
  causes of, 147–148
  complications, 149–150
bacterial lymphadenitis, acute, 209–212
bacterial sinusitis, acute, 165, 169
  amoxicillin, as firstline empiric antibiotic
    for, 165
  with standard-dose clavulanate, 166
  diagnosis, 169
  pathogen causing, 165
  treatments
    FDA approved for Augmentin XR, 170
    ostiomeatal complex, dysfunctional, 170
    for prior amoxicillin therapy, for otitis
      media, 170
bacteriuria, 3–5
Bartonella henselae, 203, 222
Bartonella quintana, 203
beta-lactam agents, 24
beta-lactamase, 87, 88
  ntHi, 89
  production, 166
black legged tick. *See Ixodes scapularis*
bladder abnormalities, 14
bocavirus, 161, 162
bony destruction, of L4-L5 vertebral bodies, 221
  radiographs, 222
Bordetella pertussis, 233
Borrelia burgdorferi, 59, 68, 69
brachial plexus palsy, 186
breast-feeding, 227
  treatment of thrush, 228
bronchiolitis, 162, 163
brown dog tick. *See Rhipicephalus sanguineus*

Campylobacter coli, 148
Campylobacter jejuni, 148
CA-MRSA. *See* community-associated
    MRSA (CA-MRSA)
CA-MRSA disease, 180
Candida albicans, 99, 227
Candida famata, 229
Candida lusitaniae, 229
Candida parapsilosis, 99, 229
Candida pulcherrima, 229
Candida tropicalis, 99
candidiasis, 43, 227, 229
  signs and symptoms of, 229

CAP. *See* community-acquired pneumonia (CAP)
cat flea. *See Ctenocephalides felis*
catheterization, 10, 11
  urine specimens, 10, 11
cat scratch disease (CSD), 207
  complicated and uncomplicated disease and
    medications, 206–207
  cultures, 204
  diagnosis of, 203
  draining sinuses and fistulas, 205
  laboratory findings, histopathology, 204
  localized, 205
  serological testing, 203
CDC. *See* Centers for Disease Control and
    Prevention (CDC)
cefixime, in children with shigellosis, 148
ceftriaxone, in treating MDR pneumococcus, 105
cell-mediated immunity, 235
Centers for Disease Control and Prevention
    (CDC), 124
  and ACOG, prevalence and prevention
    of CMV, 199
  application of pesticides to, 56
  created National MRSA Education Initiative, 36
  creating tick safe zone, 57
  prenatal CMV screening, 191
  prevention and treatment of MRSA infection, 33
  recommend 2-phased diagnostic approach, 70
  reported fatal cases of MRSA, 31
  surveillance of AGE after RotaTeq (RV5), 154
Centor score, 128
cephalexin, 18, 23, 24, 98, 114
cephalosporins
  against MSSA, 98
  nonanaphylactic allergy to, 88
  as option, for penicillin-allergic patient, 114
  resistance, 87
  in treating MDR pneumococcus, 103
cerebrospinal fluid (CSF), 189
cervical lymphadenitis, 109
chemoprophylaxis, for prevention of tick bites, 55
chemoprophylaxis, for siblings of patients with
    GAS pharyngitis, 123
children
  antibiotic options, for CA-MRSA, 24, 179
  AOM pathogen among, 87
  clinically suspected pyelonephritis, 14
  culture, with clinical signs and symptoms
    of tinea capitis, 48
  DEET in children, AAP recommendation, 56
  echocardiography, 217
  empiric therapy for, 65
  full-body skin examination, 55
  fungal load, 48
  GAS pharyngitis in, 128
  influenza-positive, 138
  intolerant/allergic to primary medications, 71
  modified Centor score, 128
  NICE approach to UTI in, 15
  oral antimicrobial therapy, 176

pneumonia in, 77–79, 165, 166
rates
    of infection in, 62
    of nasopharyngeal colonization in, 176
recommendation for Picaridin, 56
resistance rate, to fluoroquinolones, 148
risk factor for acquisition of CMV, 198
traditionally recommended antibiotic for, 67
    anaplasmosis, 61
    candidiasis, 43
    ehrlichiosis, 61
    kerion, 43
    PSGN, 119
    rotavirus disease, 154
    S aureus pneumonia, 179–181
Chlamydia psittaci, 83
Chlamydia trachomatis, 78, 81
Chlamydophila pneumoniae, 78, 175
chloramphenicol, resistance rates, 148
chlorhexidine, 27, 29
    for infection control, 29
    washes, 29
cimetidine, as prophylactic medication
    for PFAPA, 239
clindamycin, 24, 68, 87, 89, 90, 210–212
    for acute bacterial adenitis, 211
    for GAS pharyngitis, 109
    MDR pneumococcal strains susceptible to, 104
    resistance, 24
    treating MDR 19A, 104
clindamycin resistance, 24
Clostridium difficile, 147, 150
    vancomycin therapy against, 151
clotrimazole, 228
CMV infection. *See* cytomegalovirus (CMV)
    infection
Colorado tick fever, 59
common variable immunodeficiency (CVID), 235
community-acquired methicillin-resistant *S aureus*
    (CA-MRSA) strains, 179
community-acquired pneumonia (CAP), 77, 81,
    120, 175, 179
    bacterial, 175–177
        treatments, 175–177
    clinical manifestations, and epidemiology, 77
    clinical presentation, 77
    laboratory analysis, 77
    major groups, 175
    physical examination, 77
    radiographic findings, 78
    serologic testing, 78–79
    symptoms, 70
community-associated MRSA (CA-MRSA),
    27, 29, 31, 35
    antimicrobial treatment, 23
    cause of CAP, 180
    to decrease transmission in households, 35
    management, algorithm for, 25
    virulence factors, 180

contamination
    of collected specimen, 3
    cross, 150
    environmental, 35
    of fomites, 35
    otorrhea to prevent, 98
    rate, 11
    to reduce risk of, 9, 10
coronary artery abnormalities. *See* Kawasaki
    disease (KD)
coronaviruses, 233
Coxiella burnetii, 83
C-reactive protein (CRP), 237
CSD. *See* cat scratch disease (CSD)
Ctenocephalides felis, 203
cutaneous dermatophyte infections, 51
CVID. *See* common variable immunodeficiency
    (CVID)
cystic fibrosis, 234
cystitis, 6, 13, 19
cytomegalovirus (CMV) infection, 189
    assessment, for actual viral transmission
        to fetus, 190
    avidity testing, 190
    CDC recommendations, 198
    congenital, 198, 199
    culture, 189, 190
    diagnosis, 189, 190
    IVIG, for treatment, 191
    OB/GYN counsel patients on, 199
    prenatal testing, 190
    prevention, 198–199
    risk factor for acquisition, 198
    risk of seroconversion, 197
    serologies, 190
    seroprevalence to, 197
    symptoms, 198
    transmission rate, 198

DEET ((*N,N*-diethyl-meta-toluamide), 55, 56
Dermacentor andersoni, 61
Dermacentor variabilis, 61
diaper dermatitis, 227
diarrhea
    bacterial, 128
        by enteropathogenic *E coli* (EPEC), 148, 151
    empiric antimicrobial therapy, 147
        WHO recommendation, 147
    rehydration therapy, 151
DiGeorge syndrome, 160
dimercaptosuccinic acid, 15
disseminated intravascular coagulation
    (DIC), 218
DMSA scan. *See* renal scintigraphy
dog tick. *See* Dermacentor variabilis
doxycycline, 24, 65–68, 71
    for acute bacterial adenitis, 211
    in cat scratch disease, 205
D-test, 25

dysuria, 6, 13
EBV infection. *See* Epstein-Barr virus (EBV) infection
eczema, 27, 228
  bleach baths, 27
Ehrlichia chaffeensis, 61
ehrlichiosis, average annual incidence, 61
emergency rooms (ERs), 141
Enterococcus, 5
enterohemorrhagic *Escherichia coli* (EHEC), 147
enuresis, 6
environmental contamination, 35
enzyme-linked immunoassays (EIAs), 134
Epstein-Barr virus (EBV) infection, 185–186, 190, 193, 218
  neurologic complications, patient with, 186
  serologies, interpretation, 193–195; *see also* infectious mononucleosis
  steroids, role in, 185
erythema migrans, 59, 69
erm gene, 24
erythrocyte sedimentation rate (ESR), 224, 237
Escherichia coli, 221
esophagitis, 227

fevers, recurring, 233–235
fluconazole, 41–43, 228
  children with candidiasis, 43
  clinical cure rate with, 228, 229
  fungal infections, treatment of, 228
fluoroquinolones, in diarrhea, 148
folliculitis, 47
Francisella tularensis, 61, 83, 210, 212
Fusobacterium necrophorum, 166

GAS (Group A *Streptococcus*) D-test, 111
GAS (Group A *Streptococcus*) pharyngitis, 127
  clinical features, 124, 128
  diagnosis, 109, 110, 113, 124
  drug of choice, 113
  macrolide, for penicillin-allergic patient, 114
  nonsuppurative complications, 113
  role of chemoprophylaxis, 123
  scoring systems, in improving diagnostic accuracy, 128
  self-limited illness, 110, 113, 117
  treatment of, 109, 113
gastroenteritis
  acute, 153
    astrovirus infections, 154
    enteric adenovirus (EAd) infections, 154
    noroviruses (NoVs) infections, 153
  bacterial *see* bacterial gastroenteritis; epidemiology, 154
genetic periodic fever syndromes, characteristics of, 238
gentian violet, 228
glomerulonephritis, acute, 109
griseofulvin, 41, 42

for treatment of tinea capitis, 41
Group A *Streptococcus* (GAS), 24, 127, 209
  in acute bacterial lymphadenitis in children, 209
  asymptomatic siblings of patient, 123
  beta-lactam agents, active against, 24
  with intermittent otorrhea, 97
  Jones criteria for acute rheumatic fever, 118
  pharyngitis, 117, 123 (*See* GAS pharyngitis)
  pneumonia associated with, 120
  toxin producing strains of, 120
Guillain-Barré syndrome, 186

Haemophilus influenzae, 87, 93, 97, 102, 138, 159, 166, 170, 176, 233
hearing loss, 95
hematuria, 6, 10, 119
hemolytic-uremic syndrome (HUS), 149, 150
H influenzae, 166
H1N1 influenza virus rapid antigen test, 137
host defense, against microbes. *See* immunity
human granulocytic anaplasmosis, 59
human immunodeficiency virus (HIV), 229
human metapnuemovirus (hMPV), 161
human monocytic ehrlichiosis, 59, 61
  laboratory findings, 66
  signs and symptoms of, 59
  treatment, 66
human rhinovirus, 161
humoral immunity, 235
  deficiency, 159
hyperinflation, 163
hypertensive encephalopathy, 119

IgG antibodies, 190
IgM antibodies, 79, 190, 194, 203
IM. *See* infectious mononucleosis (IM)
immune system
  deficiency in, 159
  evaluation of, 235
immunity, 155, 159, 186, 198, 199, 235
immunodeficiency, 147, 229, 230, 234, 235
impetigo, 209
infections
  acute EBV, 186
  bacterial, 27, 138
  CAP in pediatric population, 175
  recurrent, 230, 233
  respiratory viral, 137
  sinopulmonary, 159
  sources, 149–150
  tick-borne, 59
infectious mononucleosis (IM), 185–186, 193
  anti-EBNA assay, 194
  anti-EBV antibodies, significance of, 195
  culture, 193
  diagnostic test, for heterophile antibodies, 194
    Monospot test, 194
  production of infectious virions, 193
  symptoms, 193

temporal kinetics, 193
inflammation
    acute, 163
    bladder, 15
    chronic, 99
    suppurative, 31
    systemic, 217
influenza, 134
influenza A and B viruses, 161
influenza diagnostic tests
    rapid respiratory syncytial virus, 135
influenza infections varies, 133
    diagnostic tests, 133
    sensitivity and specificity, 133
intensive care unit (ICU), 180
interferon gamma release assay (IGRA), 223
intermittent AOM, 87, 88, 90, 101
    no allergy to penicillin, 88
    nonsevere amoxicillin allergy/intolerance, 88
    severe amoxicillin allergy, 88
intermittent otorrhea, 97
intravenous immunoglobulin (IVIG), 191
itraconazole, 41, 42
Ixodes pacificus, 60, 69
Ixodes scapularis, 60, 67, 69

Kawasaki disease (KD), 50, 215
    clinical manifestations, 216
        coronary angiogram, 219
        two-dimensional echocardiogram, 219
    diagnosis of, 215, 219
        algorithm, 217
    drug hypersensitivity, 218
    infectious diseases causing, 218
    management, 217
    morbidity and mortality, 215
    treatment, 218
        IVIG administration, 191
KD. *See* Kawasaki disease
kerion, 43
Koplik spots, 218

Legionella, 83
Lemierre syndrome, 210
leukocyte esterase (LE), 3
linezolid, 24
lone star ticks. *See Amblyomma americanum*
low birth weight, 227
lower respiratory infection (LRI)
        symptoms, 163
lyme disease, 59, 60, 65, 67
    antibiotic treatment regimens
        for early disseminated and late lyme
            disease, 73
    cases in the United States, 59, 70
    CDC recommendation, 2-phased diagnostic
        approach, 70–71
    clinical manifestations, 61
    diagnosis of, 70
    erythema migrans rash, 70

IDSA recommendation, prophylaxis, 67
    serious manifestations of, 72
    temporally based stages, 69
lymphadenitis, 204, 212
    acute, bacterial causes in children, 209–210
    clinical features, 209
    differential diagnosis, 209
    treatments, 209–212
lymphadenitis, acute
    anaerobes, 210
    Francisella tularensis, 210
    group B *Streptococcus* (GBS), 209
    Staphylococcus aureus/Group A *Streptococcus*
        (GAS), 209
    Yersinia pestis, 210
lymphadenopathy, 6, 66, 67, 185, 193, 209, 237
lymphocytes
    EBV infecting, 185–186
    expansion of cytotoxic CD8+ T lymphocytes,
        195
    subset analysis, 160, 235

macrolides
    in atypical pneumonia, 82
    in children with hypersensitivity to
        beta-lactam antibiotics, 177
    effective in treating Lyme disease, 71
    for penicillin-allergic patient, 114
magnetic resonance imaging (MRI), 191, 222
    advantage to, 222
    vertebral osteomyelitis, 222
mastitis, 228
MDR-SP. *See* multidrug-resistant *Streptococcus
        pneumoniae* (MDR-SP)
mean inhibitory concentration (MIC), 165
measles (rubeola), 218
medical treatment failures, 100
medications
    antifungal, 228, 229
    in cat scratch disease, 206
    for early disseminated and late Lyme disease, 73
    nonsteroidal anti-inflammatory, 119
    to prevent fever episodes, 239
    side effects, 148
methicillin-resistant *Staphylococcus aureus* (MRSA),
        210. *See also* community-associated MRSA
    colonization, 27
        spread of infection, 45
    first-generation cephalosporin, 210
    messages for patient, 36–37
    occur in school, 33
    organism detected by biopsy, 222
    outbreaks in athletes, 33
    patient education, 36
    prevention of transmission, 33
    product to use for cleaning, 36
methicillin-resistant *Staphylococcus aureus*, 166, 177
methicillin-susceptible *Staphylococcus aureus*
        (MSSA), 23, 24, 29, 98, 166
metronidazole, 151

for acute bacterial adenitis, 211
Miconazole, 228
Microsporum audouinii, 51
Microsporum canis, 42, 45
middle ear effusion (MEE), culture of, 94
minocycline, 24
Moraxella catarrhalis, 97, 166, 170
MRSA. *See* methicillin-resistant *Staphylococcus aureus* (MRSA)
MSSA. *See* methicillin-susceptible *Staphylococcus aureus* (MSSA)
mucositis, 227
multidrug-resistant *Streptococcus pneumoniae* (MDR-SP), 93, 102
mupirocin
    nasal, 27, 28
    for personal hygiene, 36
    with recurrent MRSA infections, 29
Mycobacterium tuberculosis, 210
Mycoplasma pneumoniae, 78, 82, 175
    cause of atypical pneumonia, 77
    diagnostic testing, 79
    Eaton's agent, 82

nasal swabs, 134
nasopharyngeal (NP), 134, 176
natural killer (NK) cells, 235
NICE approach to UTI in, 15
NK cells. *See* natural killer (NK) cells
noroviruses (NoVs), 153
NP. *See* nasopharyngeal (NP)
nystatin, 228, 229

oral antimicrobial therapy, 176
oral candidiasis, 227, 229
    causing thrush, 227–229
osteomyelitis, 221
    diagnosis, 221
    imaging modalities, 222
    pathogens detected by biopsy, 222–223
    therapy, 223–224
    T2-weighted image, 222
otorrhea
    affinity for foreign bodies, 98
    antimicrobials and/or corticosteroids, 98–99
    chronic
        primary drug for, 98
        treating, water bugs, 99
    culture of, 98
    medical treatment failures, 97, 100
        placement of PE tubes, 97
    multidrug resistant pathogens, 98
    topical therapy, 97

pain
    abdominal, 61, 65, 66, 109, 128, 147, 149, 180, 205, 218, 238, 1545
    acute otitis media (AOM)–related, 87
    with aphthous stomatitis and

pharyngitis, 239
    breast, 228
    flank, 5, 6, 13
    low back, 221
    nipple, 228
    oral ulcers, 237
    posterior oropharynx, 237
    throat, 109, 185
parainfluenza 1, 2, and 3 viruses, 161
patients
    acute bacterial sinusitis, 165, 166
    algorithm for diagnosis with incomplete Kawasaki disease, 217
    amoxicillin treatment, 165–166, 169
    atypical pneumonia, 77–79
    cat scratch disease, 203–207
    conditions for predisposing, to recurrent infections, 229
    Escherichia coli diarrhea, 148
    erythema migrans, 59, 69
    frequent respiratory infections, 233
    with GAS, 113, 120
    high prevalence for UTI, 5, 6
    immune deficiency in, 159
    with PFAPA, 239
    on prevalence and prevention of CMV, 199
    recurrent MRSA infections, 27–29
    recurring fevers, 233–235
    sepsis evaluation, 137–138
    septicemia, 150
    severe EBV disease, 186
    skin and soft tissue infections, 32, 36
    suspected acute bacterial lymphadenitis, 209–212
    Sydenham's chorea, 117, 118
    treating MDR, 102
    with VUR, 17–18
PBPs. *See* penicillin-binding proteins (PBPs)
PCR. *See* polymerase chain reaction (PCR)
penicillin
    allergy, 88, 89, 90, 166
    for GAS pharyngitis, 109–110, 113
penicillin-binding proteins (PBPs), 165
penicillin-resistant pneumococcus, 170
periodic fever, aphthous stomatitis, pharyngitis, and cervical adenitis syndrome (PFAPA), 237–239
    with cimetidine, 239
    diagnosis of, 238
    fever pattern, 238
    genetic testing, 238
    symptoms, 238, 239
    tonsillectomy, 239
    treatment, 239
peritonsillar abscess, 109
persistent/recurrent AOM, 87, 89
amoxicillin clavulanate intolerance, 89
    drug intolerance, 89
    nonsevere amoxicillin allergy, 89
    no penicillin allergy, 89

true severe penicillin allergy, 89
PFAPA. *See* periodic fever, aphthous stomatitis, pharyngitis, and cervical adenitis syndrome
pharyngitis, 109, 110, 113, 127
  GASDirect Test, 110–111
  RADT, for initiation of therapy, 110
  sensitivity, 110
  throat culture, disadvantage of, 110
Picaridin (2-(2-hydroxyethyl)-1-piperidinecarboxylic acid 1-methylpropyl ester), 55, 56
pneumococcal conjugate vaccine (PCV), 87, 93, 101, 166, 176
pneumonia, 77–79, 165–166
polymerase chain reaction (PCR), 137, 141, 193, 207
positive rapid respiratory syncytial virus (RSV) antigen test, 142
  emergency departments (EDs), 142
  important aspects, 141
poststreptococcal glomerulonephritis (PSGN), 119
  signs and symptoms, 119
poststreptococcal reactive arthritis (PSRA), criteria for diagnosis, 119
Pott's disease, 223
Powassan encephalitis, 59
prenatal imaging, 14
prophylaxis. *See also* antibiotics
  Australian PRIVENT, findings of, 20
  doxycycline recommended drug for, 65
  GAS recommendation, 124
  in higher grade VUR, 14
    grades (III-V) of reflux, 14, 15, 19
  with penicillin/cephalosporin for, 123
  recommended dosing for UTI, 18
psittacosis, 83
psoriasis, 47, 228
pulmonary edema, 65
pyelonephritis, 5, 13, 14
pyuria, 3–5, 11

Q fever, 59, 83

rapid influenza testing, 142
rapid streptococcal antigen test, 210
  asymptomatic siblings of patient, treatment, 123–125 (*See also* GAS pharyngitis)
  throat culture, 109–111
rapid urine testing
  dipstick, 3
  microscopy, 3, 5
    vs. sensitivity of "bagged" specimen, 10
recurrent MRSA skin infection, 23–25
  bleach baths/chlorhexidine plus mupirocin ointment, 27–29
  oral antibiotic therapy, 23–25
  spread of, 31, 32, 33
renal injury, 17
renal scintigraphy, 15

acute pyelonephritis, 15
renal ultrasound, 13
  findings from urinary tract infection, 13–14
respiratory syncytial virus (RSV), 133–135, 142, 161
  antigen test, 138
  with hMPV coinfection, 163
  laboratory diagnosis, 134
    sensitivity and specificity, 133
respiratory viral illness, 138, 161, 233
reverse transcriptase-polymerase chain reaction (RT-PCR), 133
  follow-up testing, 135
RHD. *See* rheumatic heart disease (RHD)
rheumatic fever, acute, 109, 118
rheumatic heart disease (RHD), 117
rhinovirus, 161–163
Rhipicephalus sanguineus, 61
Rickettsia rickettsii, 60
rifampin, 24
RMSF. *See* Rocky Mountain spotted fever (RMSF)
Rocky Mountain spotted fever (RMSF), 59, 61, 65, 66, 218
  causative agent, 60
  in continental United States, 60
  features, 59
  laboratory abnormalities, 61
  manifestation, 60
  mortality and morbidity, 66
  primary vectors of, 61
  rash, 59, 61
  signs and symptoms, 65
  treatment, 66
Rocky Mountain wood tick. *See Dermacentor andersoni*
rotaviruses, 154–155
  common U.S. strains, 150–151
  level of efficacy, REST findings, 155
  national immunization rate, 155
  NREVSS network, 155
  strain-specific variations, 155
  types, based on capsid proteins, 155
  vaccines, effectiveness, 155

SCID. *See* severe combined immunodeficiency (SCID)
seborrheic dermatitis, 47
selective IgA deficiency, 160
selenium sulfide, as adjunctive therapy in, 41
sepsis
  due to *Yersinia enterocolitica*, 147, 148, 150
  evaluation, 137–138
  and necrotizing pneumonia, 180
septicemia, 150
serious bacterial infections (SBIs), 138
  in influenza-positive infants, 138
severe combined immunodeficiency (SCID), 229
sexually transmitted infection, 6
Shiga-toxin, 147
Shigella, 147

skin and soft tissue infections (SSTIs), 23, 32, 36
sore throat, 120
Southern tick-associated rash illness, 59
spleen, ultrasound, 205
Staphylococcus aureus (SA), 23, 27, 31, 35, 36, 94, 98,
　　120, 166, 176, 177, 179, 210, 221
　dose–response killing, 28
　epidemiology of, 31
　pneumonia, 179, 180 (*See also Staphylococcus
　　aureus* pneumonia)
　transmission, 179
Staphylococcus aureus pneumonia, 180, 181
　empiric therapy, 180
　laboratory analysis, 180
　morbidity and mortality, 180
　risk factors for, 181
　seasonal peak, 179
　and spontaneous pneumothoraces, 180
　symptoms, 176, 179
Staphylococcus epidermidis, 10, 210
Staphylococcus saprophyticus, 10
steroids
　in combination with antifungal agents, 43
　for treatment of infectious mononucleosis, 185
　　randomized-controlled trials, 185
Stevens-Johnson syndrome, 218
stomatitis, 237
stool
　colorless, 150
　culture, 142
　mucus in, 137
　watery, 148
strep pharyngitis. *See* pharyngitis
streptococcal disease
　features associated with, 129
　and presence of indicators of possible viral
　　illness, 128
streptococcal toxic shock syndrome (STSS), 120
Streptococcus pneumoniae, 77, 87, 93, 97, 103, 104,
　　120, 165, 175, 221, 233
　resistance to macrolides, 177
Streptococcus pyogenes, 102, 109, 176, 218
Streptococcus pyogenes exotoxin A (SPEA), 120
STSS. *See* streptococcal toxic shock
　　syndrome (STSS)
suprapubic catheterization, 10
Sydenham's chorea, 117, 118

TB skin test (TST), 223
T-cell immunodeficiency, 234
terbinafine, 41, 42, 44
　active against *Microsporum spp,* 42
　adverse reactions, 42
　fungicidal agent inhibiting squalene
　　epoxidase, 41
　oral course, inadequate in treating, 41
tetracyclines, 24
　for acute bacterial adenitis, 211
　adverse effects in pediatrics, 166
　recurrent MRSA skin infection, 23

third-line AOM drug, 87, 88
thrush, treatment of, 228–229
tick-borne illnesses, in North America, 59
tick-borne relapsing fever, 59
tick repellants, 55
tick safe zone, 57
tick transmission, 55
tinea capitis, 41
　antifungals for treatment, 42
　barriers to cure, 43
　cross-sectional surveillance study
　　examination, 45
　　hygiene practices, 46
　differential diagnosis, 47
　eradication of, 46
　gray-type, 47
T-lymphocyte response, 186
TM. *See* tympanic membrane (TM)
TMP-SMX antibiotic treatment, for
　　diarrhea, 151
Trichophyton mentagrophytes, 51
Trichophyton rubrum, 51
Trichophyton soudanense, 51
Trichophyton spp., 43
Trichophyton tonsurans, 42, 43, 45, 51
　genetically distinct strains, 51
Trichophyton verrucosum, 51
Trichophyton violaceum, 51
Trichophyton yaoundei, 51
trichotillomania, 47
trimethoprim-sulfamethoxazole (TMP/SMX), 24,
　　93, 148, 205, 206, 210, 211
tularemia, 59, 61, 62
　antibiotic for therapy, 67
　characterization, 59
　glandular form, common form of, 62
　　ulceroglandular lesion, 62
　incubation period, 65
　peak period of illness, 62
　reported cases in the United States, 62
TWAR agent, 82
tympanic membrane (TM), 93
tympanocentesis, 93, 94

upper respiratory infection/lower respiratory
　　infection (URI/LRI) symptoms, 163
upper respiratory tract infections (URIs), 159,
　　163, 169
urinary tract infections (UTIs), 3, 142
　antibiotics for, 18
　catheterized specimen, 9
　NICE approach, 15
urine culture, 3
　colony counts, 4
　diagnostic accuracy of rapid urine testing, 4
　problem with, 3
　for recurrent UTIs, 5
urine dipstick, 3, 5
　as rapid test of urine, 5
　vs. sensitivity of "bagged" specimen, 10

URIs. *See* upper respiratory tract
    infections (URIs)
UTIs. *See* urinary tract infections (UTIs)

vancomycin
    for acute bacterial adenitis, 211
    for children with MRSA pneumonia, 180
    intravenous agent in CA-MRSA, 24
    when metronidazole ineffective, 151
varicella zoster virus, 233
vertigo, 94
vesicoureteral reflux (VUR), 13, 15, 17–19
    bilateral, 15
    grading of, 19
    RIVUR study, 18

Vibrio cholera, 148, 150
viral capsid antigen (VCA), 194
viral respiratory infections, 161, 233
    etiology, for infants, 161
    pathogens, 161
        seasonal patterns, 161–163
voiding cystourethrogram (VCUG) test, 14, 19
voiding dysfunction, 6

Western Black legged tick. *See Ixodes pacificus*
wheezing, 163
Wiskott-Aldridge syndrome, 160

Yersinia enterocoliticar, 147
Yersinia pestis, 210

Wait...There's More!

SLACK Incorporated's Health Care Books and Journals offers a wide selection of books in the field of Pediatrics. We are dedicated to providing important works that educate, inform and improve the knowledge of our customers. Don't miss out on our other informative titles that will enhance your collection.

The exciting and unique *Curbside Consultation Series* in pediatrics is designed to effectively provide pediatricians with practical, to the point, evidence based answers to the questions most frequently asked during informal consultations between colleagues.

Each specialized book included in the *Curbside Consultation Series* in pediatrics offers quick access to current medical information with the ease and convenience of a conversation. Expert consultants who are recognized leaders in their fields provide their advice, preferences, and solutions to 49 of the most frequent clinical dilemmas in pediatrics.

Written with a similar reader-friendly Q and A format and including images, diagrams, and references each book in the *Curbside Consultation Series* in pediatrics will serve as a solid, go-to reference.

Curbside Consultation in Pediatric Asthma: 49 Clinical Questions
Aaron Chidekel MD

256 pp., Soft Cover, 2012, ISBN 13 978-1-55642-987-3, Order#79873, **$79.95**

Curbside Consultation in Pediatric GI: 49 Clinical Questions
Joel R. Rosh MD; Athos Bousvaros MD, MPH

250 pp., Soft Cover, Due: Early 2013, ISBN 13 978-1-61711-014-6, Order# 70146, **$79.95**

Curbside Consultation in Pediatric Dermatology: 49 Clinical Questions
James Treat MD

250 pp., Soft Cover, 2012, ISBN 13 978-1-61711-003-0, Order# 70030, **$79.95**

Curbside Consultation in Pediatric Infectious Disease: 49 Clinical Questions
Angela L. Myers MD, MPH

248 pp., Soft Cover, 2012, ISBN 13 978-1-61711-001-6, Order# 70016, **$79.95**

Curbside Consultation in Pediatric Ophthalmology: 49 Clinical Questions
Rudolph Wagner MD

275 pp., Soft Cover, Due: Mid 2013, ISBN 13 978-1-61711-059-7, Order# 70597, **$79.95**

Please visit **www.Healio.com/books** to order any of the above titles!
24 Hours a Day...7 Days a Week!